The Ancient Taiji Art of Lazhu Fangfa

The Ancient Taiji Art of Lazhu Fangfa

◆

The Candle Method of Taiji

Willard J. Lamb

iUniverse, Inc.

New York Lincoln Shanghai

The Ancient Taiji Art of Lazhu Fangfa
The Candle Method of Taiji

iUniverse books may be ordered through booksellers or by contacting:

iUniverse
2021 Pine Lake Road, Suite 100
Lincoln, NE 68512
www.iuniverse.com
1-800-Authors (1-800-288-4677)

Because of the dynamic nature of the Internet, any Web addresses or links contained in this book may have changed since publication and may no longer be valid.

The views expressed in this work are solely those of the author and do not necessarily reflect the views of the publisher, and the publisher hereby disclaims any responsibility for them.

ISBN: 978-0-595-45157-9 (pbk)
ISBN: 978-0-595-69540-9 (cloth)
ISBN: 978-0-595-89466-6 (ebk)

Printed in the United States of America

This book is dedicated to the sage people, those ancients instrumental in the development and perpetuation of a system of thought and fighting that is unparalleled in the martial world. In addition, I would like to thank my students for enduring the vagaries of my teaching methods.

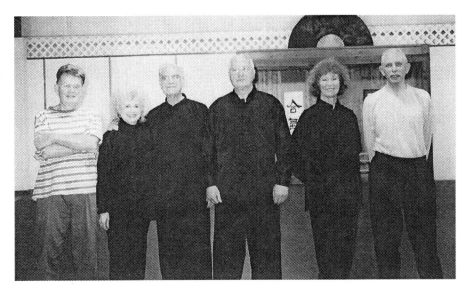

figure 1. Class photo: Left to right, Jim Lester, Evi Hartung, Rod Hartung, Laoshi Lamb, Sue Grizzard, John O'Dwyer

Contents

Section Two: Energy Storage

Section Three: Hard Jings Training

Section Four: Higher Consciousness

Acknowledgments

There are many people in this life we have been given that mold thought and behavior in us and those around us in a manner that builds constructive thought and behavior and leads us to attain what we thought only possible for more capable others. In appreciation, I would like to thank my wife, my students and all the martial artists that I have encountered and from whom I have learned much.

Introduction

Lazhu fangfa is an ancient Chinese method of training fa jin or the striking potential within the internal arts. Historically, the source of this technique resides in the fog of prehistory. Lazhu fangfa's unpretentious simplicity is its most important feature. This is completely within Taoism's belief that training can be accomplished with a surprising minimum of equipment and effort. The results of this technique are immediate and obvious and the implication of this transcends normal fighting techniques. It is an effective means for validating the efficacy of qi in training fa jin. The use of the lazhu or candle not only makes the existence of qi manifest, but it can indicate the amount of force of qi in its application.

The art of lazhu fangfa is incomprehensible to those who do not experience its subtleties. Within the traditional Chinese training methodology, only inner students train in this technique, those behind the door, and rarely is it directly taught to the public. It is not obvious to most students of Taiji that all of the things that the teachings in reference to movement within the form and fighting sequences are also true within the striking aspects of the art. Taiji is such an elegant and gracious art and yet such a confounding martial art that most individuals new to the art are not aware that the powerful forces inherent in Taiji will not spontaneously flow with no discernable effort on their part. It is certain that they will eventually flow in this manner, but this only occurs after an exceptionally long and dedicated training. Few individuals in the western society that have the determination, temperament, dedication and endurance required to sustain this life of harsh and persistent training. A long time in Taoist sense within that community means a minimum of ten years of intense training.

Lazhu fangfa is normally taught only to very few students as hui huo or hidden method in traditional Taiji. These students are only the most dedicated and morally trustworthy students, those that through the test of time and dedication have endured the incessant demands of their taskmasters. Hui hou is that secret knowledge transmitted to the few inner students that survived the elimination process. Some of this hui huo consisted of the ancient art of lazhu fangfa. Even today, there are only vague references to its existence. Most people have never seen it exhibited, and those that have seen it generally do not understand what it is they have seen. Even at its lowest level of force ming jing (visible force) the experience of lazhu fangfa takes on a mystifying atmosphere. Lazhu fangfa is only one of the overwhelming mysteries surrounding Taiji but it is by far the most disconcerting. A demonstration can inspire feelings of awe in those that witness it, and the use of these techniques in an actual physical encounter is enough to devastate most martial strategies. This book is an introduction into just one of those mysteries and it should inspire you to seek those other daunting and awe-inspiring mystic qualities of Taiji.

The Taiji of Taoism is not the Taiji that most of us practice. The teachings of Taiji do not directly express the concepts in this book. It is implied. Taoism is an experiential philosophy and does not deal in causation in the western sense of the word. This book deals with the non-traditional inferences derived from long-term study and practice of Taiji. Do not assume the ancients directly or indirectly stated these concepts, but anyone who has dealt with these forces and actually used them can attest to the viability of these precepts. What the ancients put forth was a methodology that if followed would yield amazing results. This book goes beyond the techniques and formal training into an area of thought about Taiji that is solely the author's. The true Taiji is not technique driven in that it is not a predetermined set of forms, but arrives out of the moment. It is zaren (doing what is natural for the moment).

Lazhu fangfa is not simply snuffing out a candle with a powerful and focused force. It is a collection of techniques in which the total is greater than the sum of its parts. It is greater because these combined methods of visualization, martial techniques and practice at the candle can lead to a unique interface between the ancient mind and the logical wisdom mind. It is this ancient mind that has access to formidable forces, that when directed by the wisdom mind can yield some truly startling results.

Section One:
Principles of Internal
Energy Development

1

Fundamentals of Internal Energy Storage

1 Lazhu Fangfa and Taoist Cosmology

The origin of lazhu fangfa probably lies within the energy Taiji calls local qi. This energy is the qi accumulated within the muscle groups produced when flexing muscles. It is quite possible that someone noticed the flutter of the candle flame when placing the hand close to the flame. What followed was an attempt to duplicate the effort. The key word here is effort. Since the initial extinguishing of the candle was from local qi and the depletion of local qi complete and immediate, the effort at extinguishing the candle was a futile effort. The harder they tried the less likely it was that it would work. Those who have labored at the candle can attest to the resilience of the flame. Palm strikes, punches, chops all would be futile. It would only be with the application of the principles of Taoism that results would occur. There certainly would have been some mutual reinforcement, in that Taoist principles worked and the candle in turn established the efficacy of the Taoist philosophy.

Lazhu fangfa is the embodiment of Taoist principles. It is more than candle practice. It is a tool for embedding the principles of Taoism within the soul of the practitioner. It is important to understand why these principles work in the martial arena and how western concepts of causation can assimilate them. What follows is a synthesis of ideas eastern and western in a progression that leads from the concepts of Taoism into a fully functional adept at the candle. This progression begins with the Tao.

Taiji is the physical separation from the Tao or the Great One and it becomes manifest in reality as a set of opposites. Taiji Chuan is the reconciliation of opposites. The opposites do not exist separately. They exist as complements of each other. Within each one there exists a small portion of the other so that their individual existence is entwined with their opposite. This reconciliation of opposites

3

or complements has enormous consequence for the student of Taiji. It would be just an ordinary martial art except for this one consideration.

It is out of the void that is not empty or the Tao from which these distinctions come. Taiji is the first separation and because of this separation, it is no longer the Great One or the Tao, it has become two, and this then is the noteworthy dichotomy of Taoism.

Taoism is not a religion, and it is not a philosophy. It is existential or more properly experiential in nature and therefore not an intellectual exercise. If you wish to study it, you must experience it. If you merely discuss it, then you are not experiencing it. Words have little meaning and almost no relevance when discussing Taoism. This is an essential and important part of any discourse on Taiji. The mental aspects of the discipline are what make Taiji truly unique, those ephemeral, serene, wordless moments that appear more meditative than martial. This is not unique to Taiji, but Taiji stresses these moments much more so than in other styles and the very essence of Taiji exists in this wordless world of the Tao. Taiji is about accessing this unique and mystifying existence and all the peculiarities that occur within it.

Any discussion of Taiji has to include Chinese historical thought on those distinct existential elements of humankind. A classical description of the meaning of spirit or soul and mental awareness in the Chinese system is a prerequisite to understanding the distinctions between this internal art form and the external styles.

The I Ching as presented by Lao Zu includes the terms yin and yang. The Chinese derived these concepts from the observations of the light and dark slopes of the mountains and this led to the concept of ziran or the natural order of heaven and earth. They believe that humankind resides in a unique place in the natural order of things. He resides between heaven and earth. The ancients in their thoughts about existence did not think in terms of causality. This is a concept of the western scientific mind, but it is necessary to insert causality into the fabric of the Chinese system of thought in order to understand it. The western mind does not readily comprehend the Taoist concepts in a non-causal way. It is this non-causal existence that is at the heart of Taiji and it is the source of the mystery that is Taiji. It will require some explanation so that the paradox that seems to be derived from the concepts of wei wu wei or action no action can be resolved in a coherent way that is conducive to western concepts of causality. Note that it is wei wu wei that occurs in the I Ching not simply wu wei as so commonly expressed and this distinction is important in resolving the paradox that occurs from action without action.

In the first instance, there was merely the undifferentiated Tao. It was and is a unity, the one. Taoist literature indicates that all of this natural order at the moment of the first movement, called Taiji, separates into yin and yang. This concept of opposites has become as much a part of our culture as it has in the Chinese society and most westerners readily accept the concepts.

The mystery and complexities of Taiji derive from that state of emptiness that exist within the adept when the opponent attacks and he can dissipate the incoming force with hua jing a minimum force. This existence is called wu wo or not me. In order to understand this state in the context of a non-traditional martial culture you must have an understanding of the classification of the mental aspects of existence in a Taoist sense. We can portray this simple distinction by diagraming the Tao with a division at the first movement or Taiji into yin and yang with the yin column to the right and yang in a column to the left. Yang is subdivided into chien and yin is separated into kun. Chien is the yang force or the active principle and all that are associated with it. Kun is the yin force. These complementary energies represent primal forces. The next differentiation under the yang force is human nature or xing. Kun separates into animal nature. Within this dichotomy, the Chinese historically portray two different classifications of the soul, hun or capricious soul and po the obtuse soul. The hun soul is the wisdom mind, its thoughts and desires delineate it, and it ascends at death to become shen or bright spirit. Ming is life process, the body, and it becomes gui or a ghost at death and po then returns to the earth

To clarify this, hun divides into the yi mind or wisdom mind and the xin mind or emotional mind. This division is a simplification of Chinese thought, but these three concepts are the foundation of Taiji training. It is necessary to discuss them in detail, even if necessary, at the expense of other concepts that are not as pertinent to this discussion.

A fundamental tenet within the Taoist cosmology is the belief that at birth the natural order encompasses two separate and unique souls or spirits and that this separate existence resides in two different realms of reality. These realms are existential in nature. They are existential in the sense that they are the result of our unique experiences and our free interaction with the natural order or ziran. Included within these features is human nature and that of animal nature. These discriminations are essential in arriving at an understanding of the structures and interplay of energies in the internal arts especially Taiji.

The Chinese designate these two realms of existence or spheres of influence as ming and xing. Within the classification designated as ming by the Chinese, resides po the spirit essence. It is the animal nature or animal spirit. Ming is, within the Chinese concept of reality, considered as life or as life process. This separation into a dichotomous existence between ming and xing is a process, an organic and living process. These two distinct existential realities entwine and interact, in the interplay of dominance, submission and even cooperation that is unique and with specific training; these separate existential realities can become increasingly interactive. The Taoists hold the belief that we begin life in this world with these two separate modes of existence, the hun spirit and the po spirit, and that there is a predetermined interplay between hun and po. Hun, the spirit exists within the human condition or xing and it separates into two aspects. They are the yi mind (the rational mind) and the xin mind (the emotional mind). It is the internal martial artist intent to momentarily exclude the xin mind and its emotional baggage and logical content of the yi mind from the martial arena by stilling the mind (yi ting shi) while at the same time maintaining a parallel existence between the yi mind (rational logical mind)and that of po (the animal mind). This unique coexistence is the subject of most of the mental training within Taiji.

Taiji is the first separation from the Tao. This unique coexistence characterizes the separation of the Tao into yin and yang. Yang is the active, masculine principle and conversely yin is the dark, inactive, feminine principle. Po is in control of the source of energy interaction between the phenomenal world and the world of po or spirit world. It stands on the edge of these worlds and it can look from its intermediate position into the phenomenal world, which consists of the world of the ten thousand things or hun, and it can look into the spirit world or the world of po. It is nonverbal, non-logical, and non-emotional. It operates within a geometry of its own contrivance. The geometric orientation of incoming and out going energies organizes its world, and it regulates these energies for life-giving reasons. It also manipulates these energies at the indirect discretion of the ego-mind or yi mind. It is in the unique position of being able to operate within both worlds with respect to the physical body and its energy system. Xing represents human nature. We know this existence as the self and all that it sees and with which interacts. It is the phenomenal world, the world of the ten thousand things or yiwan dongxi as the Chinese call the world in which we live.

Existence within the realm of po is to experience primitive perceptions of the energies that exist within daily life. The world of hun does not directly experience these energies. These are the life-giving energies and the human nature aspects of ming. Ming and xing are existential categories created by the separation of our existence into the yin and yang of the first movement or existential separation. These dichotomies exist because of this separation. This is an evolutionary development of the two systems and the reality of this separation exists within the use of words and the logical arrangements of them. Po does not use words, but engages this existence in a more primal and symbolic manner. It interacts directly with the body in order to deal with the energy requirements of the body. It has the ability to manipulate the body but does not ordinarily move the body within the world of the ten thousand things. Within the complexities of the ordinary world, po is a trance like state unless trained. It is reactive, monitors the conditions around it, and makes adjustments accordingly. It does not react to concepts of past or future, but training to receive information of the world of the ten thousand things from the yi mind and to act on it is possible accordingly. There is a qualitative difference between existence within po and the yi mind. The paralyzing fear that debilitates most of us in an altercation is the result of the yi mind utilizing its knowledge of past and future and then escaping the conflict because of this excessive fear. This leaves behind an untrained po. It is untrained in the sense that it does not react to the phenomenal world in the normal sense. Existence is a continuum that consists of maximum ego-involvement or yi mind at one end to the maximum noninvolvement or trance-like-states of po on the other hand. It is within these maximum trance-like-states that maximum control and maximum use of those exotic and esoteric internal forces come into play. It is this interplay of the yi mind in the world of the ten thousand things and the mind of po within its energy matrix that the mysteries of Taoism become known.

The concept of the Sage in Taoist philosophy involves this cognitive internal exchange between yi and po. There are specific things, which will automatically place the zhenzhung ren, the observer, or the immortal as the Chinese call it; the literal translation is real or genuine human, within the world of po and not hun. There are mental disruptions in which the wisdom mind or hun, the yi mind aspect, seeks to escape from the perceived reality of imminent death. Serenely straddling the cusp of this line between imminent death and safety is the intent of the warrior, and this distinguishes his unique essence. It is this immediate access to po that the warrior seeks. Without specific training, po continues to monitor the energy system, oblivious to any non-energy-oriented threat within the phenomenal world. The trance is a state of monitoring the body. This is a neutral condition and po waits for a change in conditions that may need modification. In this sense, death is the ally of the warrior mind. It can use the yi mind's fear of death to allow access to po. The yi mind's propensity to escape fearful situations is the key to access to po. This bears repeating; the yi mind's natural inclination to escape a fearful encounter is the means of access to po.

Hun, which is the opposing yang aspect comparable to ming, which is yin, occupies the phenomenal world, the world of the ten thousand things. The first movement, within the original undifferentiated state of Tao, is a separation into yin and yang. The principles of non-action and action, dark and light, no and yes that everyone is familiar with have become a part of our culture, as well as the Chinese culture.

The nature of po is such that it operates within the "eternal now." It does this because it has no concept of past or future. It does not manipulate concepts such as past and future in the usual sense. It manipulates geometric relationships or visualizations. Past, present and future are concepts within our minds, they do not exist in the direct encounter with the world, as po perceives it. Po is concerned with moving energy to and from the body and moving the body around the obstacles of the world. It is also concerned with life-giving processes and the manipulation of energy for those purposes. In order to manipulate energy, po must envision it directly and interact with it directly. It does this in a manner much different from hun. It is by understanding the ways in which po manipulates energy that we can make use of these energies and develop them for martial purposes. Manipulating these energies and the resultant effects on the relationship between po and hun is the reason martial artist considers their art as a road to enlightenment and the Tao.

1-2 Theory of the Soft and Yielding

One major difference that separates the external style and the internal style of the martial arts and illustrates a critical departure in philosophy is the means internal artist handle incoming force. The external style uses force against force as seen in a forceful blocking maneuver or direct attack. This method uses large striated muscle groups, and the amount of energy expended is extremely high. The internal styles, on the other hand, will intercept an incoming fist in a circular manner so that the interception is at a point in which the hand of the adept is moving in the same direction as the incoming force. This allows the interception to be almost imperceptible. If the opponent is not aware of your interception, it is then possible to move him and manipulate him out of his original line of direction so that he misses you. He will discover only visually that he has missed you. The strategic relevance of this error lies in the fact that he will have to discern visually that he has missed. The reason he has missed will not be evident to him and this will immediately destroy his strategy. It is a strategy, which has served him effectively in most other situations. It has not been successful in this situation, he cannot ascertain the reason, and it will not be immediately evident to him. Between the moment of the missed strike and his conscious awareness of it, exists considerable time and opportunity for the adept. There is much energy conserved by this method and this has martial value.

After the initial strike by the opponent, you can follow his strike in the direction it was going, or you can add energy to his withdrawal and manipulate him in either direction. The act of following and adding additional energy to his movement requires little effort on your part and can be devastating to him. By yielding to the opponent, you also can allow him to move into a position to your advantage and push through his center to uproot him. Yielding can also effectively allow you to lead by walking away. You can lead him into emptiness (yin jin luokong) by moving him and taking away his prop when he is unbalanced. Manipulating the individual in more than one direction at a time can have a devastating effect on his ability to maintain his root. Probably the most powerful, yet seemingly innocuous techniques involve using whole body power. They are devastating because they occur without warning and so rapidly that it is not possible to defend against them. With fa jin, you are disengaged and there is a short time interval between the inception and conclusion of the strike. With whole body power, direct contact with the individual reduces the time interval. When the opponent uses force against force, he is telegraphing his connection and his intention. You can then adjust to his force. When your touch is soft (rou), it is then possible to understand the intentions of the opponent. You can therefore manipulate, divert and assist his movement in a deliberate and considerate manner. The circular movement from yin to yang is a characteristic of Taiji. The form and actual combat is always interplay between various degrees of maximum and minimum force (gang and rou). It is offensive then defensive, yin then yang until the opponent is dealt with through fa jin or some other technique. Other styles over extend and become unbalanced, they emphasize the yang portion of the sinusoidal wave of force and you should note that this sinusoidal wave is a circular function, and Taiji always moves in a circular manner. Taiji emphasizes the yin portion of the wave and instead of initiating the action, it begins with the yielding, soft and yin portion of the sinusoidal wave of energy by intercepting and then setting up for the peak spike of energy that represents fa jin or an jing, and then to immediately revert back to the soft and yielding.

Manipulation of the opponent's awareness of your contact to your advantage when you grasp the concept of the soft is possible. Appear and disappear in a manner that confuses your opponent becomes possible. You can then lead him with a light touch of the hand. The options presenting themselves using the soft techniques are incredible when compared to using force against force.

The soft and yielding are not relevant concepts within the martial arts community and are not natural to the external martial art. It takes a great deal of faith in ones ability to handle the opponent to accept the concept that in the martial arena, the soft can overcome the hard and that the weak can overcome the strong. It is even more difficult for the external styles to accept this, because they have considerable investment in using the strong, the fast and the hard. Normal everyday experience seems to reinforce the concepts of the external styles. It is easy to hold the concepts of the soft in an intellectual manner, but we all revert to the hard when confronted by an immediate threat. It requires operating from some mental level other than the ego in order to operate in a soft and yielding manner. It becomes a matter of training the mind, in order to enter this peculiar state of mind the Chinese martial artist call po. This state is part of the animal nature of man. This is the ancient mind and represents the primitive aspect.

At this point, the student trains in a three-pronged approach to every technique. They train the soft and yielding in conjunction with po as a component of the technique.

This triad, consisting of po, visualizing the soft and yielding, and the techniques, is inherent in the methodology of training, especially the visualization techniques. The training techniques for the soft and yielding are unique to the internal arts and the key is to treat the incoming energy indifferently, avoiding the emotional charge or xia qi that results from an assault on our senses. Be serene and do not react to xia qi. It is by relegating the assault to a concept of moving energy, devoid of social context, that we can neutralize it effortlessly. The minute it becomes something other than moving energy, we react to it violently and enter the arena of the hard (gang). To maintain the soft, it is necessary to use some trigger in the sequence of events prior to the release of the incoming energy that will initiate the esoteric state of po. This mental state is a prerequisite to functioning in a soft and yielding manner. The triggering mechanisms will be detailed later on in another chapter.

1-3 Relaxation

The conventional definition of relaxation is not the definition used in Taiji. In the martial sense, relaxation is a tension reduction that yields an extended endurance over considerable time. This ability to extend our capabilities beyond normal endurance characterizes this technique. Even when actively doing something, it is an enduring event sustainable overtime until terminated. This acquired endurance is a result of the ability to support whatever activity is on going at the time and use no more effort than is required to sustain it.

The Indians of the Andes run scores of miles at high altitudes in a steady rhythmical manner, which appears to be an effortless accomplishment considering the conditions. They are capable of reducing the inner tensions that most of us have, so that they do not waste energy or hinder their efforts. To function effectively at extreme heights the significantly reduced oxygen level requires even more effort for the uninitiated to function at this level. This is more than mere acclimation to different conditions. It is a cluster of physiological functions that most of us cannot duplicate.

The Japanese warriors in their canoes could row rhythmically for hours without tiring. Within the Japanese martial arts today exists a rowing exercise. It is a combination of breathing and standing rowing movements that mimic the ancient ways. It builds endurance through breathing and relaxation within a rhythmical movement. This allows one to mentally wait, and put mental effort on hold until the end of the discipline.

The form in Taiji is a medium for developing this relaxed effortless combination of breathing and rhythmical behavior that leads to reduced tension and consequently to increased endurance. The Taiji form takes the individual into a different level of consciousness, which facilitates this endurance so critical to martial endeavor. Practice the form with the opponent visualized as if he stood before you in each individual stance. This meaningful relationship with the imagined adversary impresses itself on po and results in training of this aspect of the mind each time you do the form.

Relaxation in the Taiji sense then becomes a relaxed state of sentience, in which the individual maintains a warrior sense of the immediate and present danger, yet is capable of sustained tension reduction that increases endurance. This sentience is unique to this particular relaxation. It is existence within the eternal now, an awareness of everything going on, without an active participation in it. This sentience is waiting without becoming engrossed in the ongoing rhythmical activity. It is a training, which will allow this tension reduction, but it is a specific type of mental training. This relaxation training is a triad in the same sense that the soft and yielding training is a triad. Soft and yielding have to do with the handling of incoming and outgoing energy, while relaxation has to do with bodily movement and the use of the musculature. To be relaxed is to move the body as if wafted by a gentle summer breeze. It is the yin side of the omnipresent yin and yang sinusoidal wave of energy and body movement. There are specific techniques, which enhance the relaxation of the body even when under extreme pressure to perform. Breathing techniques, opening and closing techniques, visualizations, and song all contribute toward this sentient relaxation.

1-4 Song

In order to utilize song (pronounced shoong), it is necessary to understand the concept. Song is not your everyday state of relaxation. It also is not an altered state of mind, but instead song is a deceptive means of avoiding tension. It is an attempt to deceive the rational mind or yi mind in its attempt to control the use of force by muscular efforts or li. It is important to use deception because of the natural tendency of the yi mind to defeat any attempt at emitting force by means other than li or external muscular effort. We always revert to external force because we have a lifetime of successful use and fear always takes us back to the basics when we are truly uncomfortable. It is necessary then to allow fear to take us to a place other than this fearful state within the yi mind.

In any discussion of Song, it is necessary to include po. The commingling of the two results from our inherent tendency to revert to the fundamentals as we learned them when confronting our worst fears. It is necessary to train ourselves to revert to this state of po in order to by pass our natural tendencies to use li.

These are soul-changing experiences that repeatedly occur throughout one's life. These are shifts in perception that transform. For instance, it would not seem possible that the simple act of looking at stars through a telescope could be one of those transforming events. It is more than a paradigm shift, which is an intellectualized model; it is an experiential shift in perspective. It is one in which you react to your perception differently and your world is rearranged to meet this adaptation. For instance, in viewing the stars through a telescope the star will track across the field of vision in the telescope and this shift in perception from the star moving to the real perception that you are moving instead can be such that the shift in orientation can cause you to become unbalanced and overcompensate for the perceived change. This compensation can be such that you can nearly flip yourself onto the ground. This is similar to the moving train phenomena in which you perceive your own stationary train as moving when another train passes and can be viewed through the windows of the compartment. Song is actually the reverse from this situation. You are actually correcting an error in the previous perceptual error.

Song when properly perceived is one of these experiential perceptual shifts that can be overwhelming and lead to insights and more importantly different ways of reacting to the physical environment.

The Chinese word that most unambiguously defines Taiji is simply song. Song is unique among concepts. Its meaning is a complex of manipulations that deftly move the Taiji adept into a state of being, a state of existence that is unique and perhaps one avoided by most people including most other martial artists. It is a state in which the yi mind has lost control, and it is a shared experience and a shared responsibility. The yi mind does not share well. It is not a team player and reserves all things to itself. This is why I say song is a complex set of manipulations.

These manipulations are in the nature of devices used to trick the body and the mind into a mental and physical state of cooperation between the yi mind and po. It is necessary to trick the yi mind because of its propensity to maintain its usual control at all cost. This cooperation is important because it is from po that the internal martial forces are derived. In order to access these forces, it is necessary to access po. The situation becomes complicated because po does not interact with the environment in a cognitive way. It is reactive in that it monitors the environment and interacts with incoming and outgoing energy. It can be trained, and this is a benefit derived from the use of song. Po can be trained to operate at the discretion of the yi mind.

Desire is the most difficult aspect of the yi mind to control. If you cannot delay gratification, then you will never be entirely song.

The word most often heard in the community of Taiji is song (shoong). You must be song. This concept is central to Taiji. It is central to the understanding of internal concepts. The knowledge of this concept is pivotal to the discovery of the power generated by the internal martial arts. Song can be defined as the ability to move the body with only minimal use of the musculature of the body. Song occurs as a result of using smooth muscle, tendons, ligaments, fascia and a host of other tissues to move the body and to move the internal energy. It is the attachment point of the long muscles, the tendons and the connection of the joints through ligaments that most people associate with movement. The fact that energy can be stored in the fascia is foreign to most of us. The fascia is a tissue support system that protects the organs of the body. The vascular system and its smooth musculature also are capable of considerable hydraulic pressure and functions indirectly in producing force. There are means of developing not only hydraulic, but also pneumatic pressure for martial purposes. Song is a highly complex issue within Taiji. It has many facets and considerable combinations.

The acceleration of the internal punch is based on the inner and outer circles of rotation. This acceleration is caused by the increase in the radial distance of the fist from the body. The farther from the body the fist is, the greater the angular momentum. The external styles also apply these principles of angular momentum. The difference is in the application of song. In the external styles, the musculature moves the arm and the fist. Within the internal styles, movement is driven by the turning of the waist and the movement of the body using whole body power in both storage and emission of energy. The arm and fist are pulled by the attachment at the shoulder and the musculature is merely a support mechanism. The components of the internal punch are very complex and will be reviewed later, but for purposes of clarifying song, it must be understood that much of the posture requirements of Taiji are actually to facilitate song.

The tilting of the hips forward results in a straightening of the spine at the ming men (hollow of the back) and this in turn facilitates the rotation of the spinal column. The unimpeded rotation of the spine is critical to song. Any tilt of the spinal column results in muscular support, which is detrimental to the proper practice of song. The forward thrust of hips in fa jin keeps the head level and oriented properly with forward movement, it also keeps the spine in balance, much as a juggler would balance a stick by moving and maintaining the hand under it.

When it is said in the classical Taiji literature that the waist governs the qi, it is in essence telling you to be song and power your movement with the waist and not the musculature. To be song is to balance your movement and move in an effortless manner maintaining your center with very little muscle involvement. Moving the waist instead of using muscles to control the movement is one of the most difficult principles of Taiji for the beginner. It is something that must be worked on constantly.

You are not entirely song if you have not developed the capacity to relax the vaso-constrictors of the arterial system. If the arterial system is constricted, then there is reduced blood flow, which interferes with the energy system and the healing properties of the body. To be completely song, you must then also relax the vaso-constrictors. This is dealt within later chapters. It relates to the unusual state of existence that is called po.

Much that is done within Taiji is accomplished by techniques that fool the body and deceive the ego mind. One important aspect of song is the utilization of a specific breathing sequence, which is contrary to normal everyday rationale. We normally hold our breath or exhale on exertion to assist in the application of force. Within Taiji, there is the concept of opening and closing, and specific breathing patterns that accompany it. Opening (movement of the extremity away from the body) should be accompanied by inhaling and closing (movement toward the body) should be accompanied by exhaling. This assists in creating a relaxed state as you emit energy as in fa jin and this allows the qi to flow. It is difficult to exert force when you are inhaling. Many of the strange or unorthodox methods of Taiji are of this nature, in which the body is tricked into being song by the techniques of training. There is a distinction between sentient relaxation and song. Relaxed sentience is the conservation or economy of movement that leads to long-range endurance. Song is utilizing different structures than the normal musculature in the body to transport the body and its posture in a martial way.

If you think in terms of song as a means of tricking the body so that a minimal li or muscular force is used it will make more sense. Song is a not a condition. It is a methodology. It is a means of causing the body to perform in a certain way that allows the intrinsic forces that exist within the body to move in prescribed ways. It is a method of removing the yi mind and its habitual way of dealing with force and substituting something else. All of those peculiarities of Taiji that make it distinct and separate it out from the external and other internal styles are due to these efforts at being song so that the energies of Taiji will freely move so they can be used in a martial sense. I must add one additional factor, which is important to song. This is the utilization of breathing during fa jin, specifically inhaling on emitting force. This is contrary to all that has been exhorted on the striking arts. Everyone knows that you exhale on exertion. This is axiomatic and part of the lore of all sports and especially the martial arts. What we do know, from the external styles and all other forms of force, is that exertion and exhaling go together. This is understandable when you are using li or muscular force to generate power. The internal arts, however, only minimally use li. If you inhale on exertion to deliver then you can be song during fa jin. This does not violate the principle that you exhale on exertion because exhaling is a simple release from inhaling, not a forceful release, but simply a cessation of inhale. This allows you to be song on the storage phase as well as the emission phase of fa jin, and at the precise moment of the release of energy you are still song and gently exhaling. The analogy of the difference between a fire and an explosion is appropriate. It is merely a difference in duration. The fire is the same amount of energy spread out over a longer period of time. What we have done is narrowed the release time or compressed it into just an instant and then we release the same amount of energy. The results can be staggering. We will discuss this in more detail later.

1-5 The Taiji Sphere

The Taiji sphere is a mental construct. It does not exist in reality. It is a mental expedient, a way of looking at the body that alters the underlying assumptions that normally prevent the postural stability, which exists in the rooting techniques of Taiji. Taiji techniques follow these principles, which are hidden within the movement of this conceptual sphere. When a martial force is exerted on the center of this sphere, these principles come into play. If a force is applied on a line drawn from the point of contact and passes through the center of the sphere, it will cause the sphere to move directly backwards. If you push on the sphere at a point in which the direction of force does not move through the center, the sphere will then rotate and move away at an angle to the force direction.

This is the fundamental principle of the sphere in Taiji. A spherical object moves with its stability and connection point in direct contact with the ground. It is rooted on this one point, and as force is exerted, it continually moves from this one point on the sphere to another point of contact. It continually moves away from this force never allowing it to penetrate into the sphere. Its inherent stability lies in the fact that it will move to another point on the sphere to maintain this stable configuration. The Taiji sphere is similar in that it moves using the substantial leg, and it moves from one rooted leg to the other continuously, to either move away or rotate the waist to prevent the force from penetrating.

Rotating the waist is an important feature in fa jin. It is also an important function in the defensive moves of the Taiji sphere. The Taiji sphere is different from an actual sphere in that it does not move away from the incoming force unless forced to, but instead moves that force around it by rotating on its one point. If, however, the incoming force is too great, then the Taiji adept moves to another point on the sphere and the insubstantial leg becomes the substantial one.

The stability of the sphere results from the movement of the central axis (the spine) and the balance of this axis over the substantial leg. This central column of the spine and substantial leg as an axis allows one to both rotate the incoming force around this central axis, but also allows one to move the one pointed base in any direction to compensate for excessive incoming force.

1-6 Stance Training

There are some fundamental differences in the performance of various stances in the internal arts that require some emphasis. This difference is evident in the manner in which the adept moves in Taiji. The spine is held in a vertical manner for several reasons. The primary reason is to prevent tension and muscle strain evident in supporting the spine at an angle. This would require the use of the long striated muscles, which would have to support this off center load. Much of the stress and strain creating back problems is of this nature. To avoid back muscular problems or compressed disc problems, you should always maintain a vertical spine. When the Taiji adept strikes with fa jin, the spine is kept vertical, if it is not, then with the arm perpendicular to the spine the distance it can reach is reduced. To maintain the same distance, you would have to extend the arm at an angle other than ninety degrees between the arm and the spine. This would reduce the effect of the acceleration due to the movement outward of the fist on a shorter radius.

The hips are pivoted forward in Taiji which has the effect of straightening the spine by reducing the curvature of the spine at the ming men point. It is located in the curvature of the small of the back. The ming men point in Chinese translates as the gate of life and it is one of the more difficult areas of movement in the transport of qi. This posture has the unified purposes of facilitating the rotation of the spine by establishing a more vertical and straight rod, and it facilitates the transport of qi through this difficult channel.

The spine is also straightened by moving the chin backward to remove the curvature at the cervical area. This creates an alignment of the spine from the perineum all the way to the head. It makes the rotation of the central spine much more liable to change by reducing tension and strain resulting from an off balanced system. The unique and unconventional look of Taiji is mostly due to the juggling movements used to maintain this balance of a vertically erect spine. It is much like a juggler trying to balance a long rod on the palm of his hand, where every movement is calculated to stay directly beneath the rod and keep it from becoming unbalanced (see figure 2).

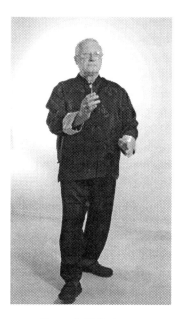

figure 2. Taiji stance

The Taiji ready stance is a perfect illustration of this balancing act. It is one of the classical requirements in formal stance training. It is the preferred posture when confronted by an external threat. The reason for this is that this particular stance contains all those things needed to enhance the proper movement when challenged. The stance is created from a ma pu posture in which the feet are a shoulder width apart and in line. You then rotate your body to the right so that the right leg is the forward one and move your center of balance so it is centered over the rear leg. Raise the forward foot so that the heel is just touching the ground, and then move your right hand to the center line of the body in a position just forward of the sternum, palm facing inward. Location of the hand in the strongest and most effective position on your center is determined by drawing a line along the anterior portion of the shin of the rear leg, and where this line intersects the line drawn horizontally from the sternum outward on your center-line is the location of the hand. The hand should be yu nu shou, the beautiful lady's hand which is a graceful curve from fingertips to the shoulder. Yu nu shou translates as jade lady's hand. This (yu nu) or jade lady is a common Chinese expression for a beautiful lady.

The spine must be vertical with the chin tucked and the ming men point must be straightened. The tongue is placed on the palate just behind the front teeth.

This serves to transfer energy in fa jin through the head without the snapping motion of the head, which is characteristic of karate and other external style punches. This snapping of the head results in tension in the shoulder area, which would be necessary to stabilize the head, and this increased tension in the shoulders restricts bodily movement and the movement of qi. Any excess tension is contrary to the principles of Taiji. This requires tension reduction to increase stamina, facilitate sensing, and to enhance the flow of qi.

In the ready stance, it is necessary to raise the shoulders and hollow the chest. Taiji literature contains many suggestions of this. The purpose is one of energy storage in preparation for fa jin or an jing. Hollowing the chest allows one to open from a closed position as in opening and closing techniques. In this instance it allows for more movement in the opening to facilitate the acceleration of withdrawal as in the technique lu, or as energy storage in the technique an. Raising the shoulders allows the spine to move in a whip like sinusoidal wave that coordinates with the forward thrust of the hips in fa jin. This movement alone can greatly facilitate the explosive power of fa jin.

The ready stance should be practiced as an immediate response to a threat. The raising of the forward foot, to a heel position, forces the center of gravity over the rear leg, and automatically creates the one pointed stance of the Taiji sphere. The arm and hand are in the beautiful ladies hand position, centered and at the most effective distance to intercept or strike. Energy is stored by raising the shoulders and hollowing the chest. Both defensive and offensive elements exist in the posture, and as in all stances pre positioning and placement of extremities is paramount.

1-7 Rooting Basics

Taiji is an internal martial art and as such, it intercepts incoming energy primarily with soft techniques and not the hard and linear blocking type of interceptions that characterize the external styles. The extremity that intercepts this incoming energy flows with the incoming energy in the direction it is moving and displaces or otherwise manipulates that energy. It is defensively oriented, and therefore utilizes soft blending techniques to set up for hard or soft offensive techniques. The energy is maneuvered around the center of this stable base formed by a rooting technique that enables one to both receive energy and deliver energy from the same stance. It is this instantaneous change from soft to an explosive hard energy and back again to a soft receptive technique that is so characteristic of Taiji, and this is fundamental to its esoteric nature. It is this rhythmic alternation from yin to yang in a continuous flowing-river-like manner with eddies and accelerations that has inspired the comparison of Taiji to the never-ending-flow of a river. The body flows as a result of moving from one rooted stance to another. Song allows the upper body to quickly turn on its axis, and rotate without losing balance or fixating on the hard. It is the Taiji sphere moving from one point of contact to the next, softly, gently and yielding as it exhibits song in a slow but forceful movement of irresistible forces that combine to move any obstacle out of its path. This apparent irresistible force is what characterizes Taiji.

Rooting can be best understood when you realize that it is independent of the direction in which the energy is moving. Force may be incoming or outgoing. When you practice rooting to handle incoming force, you are also training to handle outgoing forces. You should note that the borrowing energy that you receive and deliver back to the opponent, has the same feel as fa jin energy. It is also true that when you practice fa jin, then you are also training to receive incoming energy. It is by way of the same channel that both energies occur.

To be able to maintain an effective root, the ground must be sensed and the contact felt under your feet. You must clench the ground with the toes. The legs are contracted as if grasping the ground. This places the yongquan point directly in contact with the surface. The yongquan is a point on the center of the ball of the foot. It is this point that is pressed in fa jin to initiate the pulse of energy that is eventually emitted at the fingertips. It helps when beginning this practice to exert an excessive amount of force in rooting, then gradually over time release the exertion until a minimum amount of energy is used, during which you can still feel this rooting sensation that maintains contact with the ground. This sensation can be enhanced by pushing against a wall or by having someone test your stance by pushing against you.

Much of the training in Taiji is based on this sensation or feeling of being rooted, and this particular connection and movement of energy within the body is something that constantly encouraged in a manner other than the normal training. These specific sensations are deliberately promoted with every practice. They must be specifically trained in a conscientious manner. You must not assume that just because you have felt the connection initially that you are successfully rooted. Much faulty training in Taiji will be because of the assumption that you are rooted. You must deliberately and constantly train yourself to be aware of this root and sustain it as you perform every movement and every technique. Your mind must be centered on the tantien (yi shou tantien), but peripherally you must sense the rooting sensations at all times.

1-8 Double Weighted Stances

The equal balance of your weight on both feet in Taiji is called double weighting. This is considered a fault and must be eliminated. This violates the principle of the Taiji sphere. You have lost the one point of balance. You also have lost the ability to move rapidly from one point of contact in your stance to another. It is conceivable that neither the forward nor the rear foot is grounded and rooted properly such that you cannot correctly apply a technique or fa jin. This means that the opponent can find a line in which to push you, one that you cannot recover from and you may be uprooted.

The training in rooting creates a position of strength for you. The opponent may be stronger and faster, but if you have the stronger root then you have the superior position. If you are able to lead him from your one stable root to another, then by moving while rooted you are moving in strength and he is vulnerable. Double weighting should be avoided at all costs, except in the momentary transition from one rooted stance to another.

The ready stance in the peng position is a practice that can be utilized to train in avoiding double weighted stances. The raised forward foot, with only the heel resting on the ground will force you to sit over the rear leg and maintain the Taiji sphere with its one point contact with the ground. It is essential that you learn to move from any given stance into another without hesitation, and be able to fa jin from that stance. Even defensive postures should yield the potential for fa jin.

1-9 Substantial and Insubstantial

The weight distribution between the forward and rear foot is usually stated in some ratio such as seventy-thirty or sixty-forty, with the substantial leg specified as the higher number. The terms substantial and insubstantial relate to the proportions of the body mass carried by each respective leg. It is important to pay particularly close attention to substantial and insubstantial in the early stages of training. The ability to move smoothly and effortlessly from one posture to another while maintaining level head height is essential. With careful attention to substantial and insubstantial, balance and posture improves. Differentiation between substantial and insubstantial allows one to take careful consideration of mass distribution as you move through the forms. Instead of floating in an unbalanced way, a deliberate one-point centering can be maintained so that the concept of the Taiji sphere is maintained throughout the practice of the form.

1-10 Posture and Its Relation to Energy Storage

The Taiji form has a considerable number of methods for storing energy and releasing it. The smooth flow of the form rounds out these break points or spikes in energy discharge or fa jin and it reduces the storage end of the sequence to an imperceptible change in direction or posture. This is not a defect in strategy because it is to your advantage to conceal your intentions; however, it is difficult for the beginner to discern those points of storage and the methods of storage.

An jing is the Chinese term for the soft jings that derive from the smooth flow of qi through the postures. These occur naturally and need little amplification. One of the significant forms of an jing that occur within the Taiji form is push or an. This is a segment of grasp the sparrows' tail. The initial movements are a withdrawal of both arms as if the hands were being drawn over a large ball. This gives a serpentine look to the withdrawal. When the hand reaches the top of the imaginary ball, the hand and arm do have a definite snake like appearance to them. In combination with this snake like movement, hollowing the chest and raising the shoulders should give this same serpentine look to the spinal column, and this occurs as the hands reach the lower portion of their withdrawal, at which time there is a natural hollowing of the chest and raising of the shoulders. In both techniques, energy has been stored in the curvatures of the structures. The pulse of energy goes through two sine waves to reach the palms in fa jin. The first pulse is at the spine and the second is in the arms. There occurs, one after another, the release of the energy of this sine wave, and it accumulates in an additive way to yield high energy. In order to avoid confusion, it is necessary to understand that the term an in Chinese has two meanings. One meaning is push and the other is hidden or secret. In both instances, the tonal is descending.

1-11 The Breath

Taiji starts with the opening stance facing north to gain from the yin forces that cool and calm what would normally be an excited state. This has a calming effect on the mind that is sought in Taiji. Every activity within the art of Taiji is performed to enhance this calm serene effect on the mind. The breath is no exception and should be yin in nature. It must cool the body and quiet the mind. It must flow smoothly and quietly, so that it does not interfere with this calming and serene effect. It must instead exhibit this feeling of stillness.

Draw the breath inward in a thin, even and delicate line of breath. How thin a stream is required can be determined by the cool feeling that you get at the moist tip of the tongue. If you are not feeling this cooling effect on the tip of your tongue, then the stream of air is not thin enough.

The breath should be delicate enough that it can only be felt on the tip of the tongue. It should be like a gentle breeze, barely perceptible. The chest muscles are not used in breathing. One of the main difficulties people have in breathing under duress is that the intercostal rib muscles contract and even go into spasms, making it very difficult to inhale. If you train yourself to breathe using the diaphragm, the tightness of the chest can be avoided and an additional benefit is that you can conceal your breathing. Experienced martial artists can key on your breathing and anticipate your actions.

While you are doing the form on occasions other than fa jin and an jing then the method of breathing should be that of Buddhist breathing. The breathing should be done with the diaphragm in such a manner that the abdomen is expanding on inhale. To facilitate placing your attention on the tantien a minimal amount of reverse Taoist breathing should be utilized so that an awareness of the tantien area is foremost in your mind. This can be accomplished by offering resistance to the abdominal expansion in a way that does not interfere with the smooth flow of the breath, but creates a sensation of tightness. This will keep the mind centered there and keep the tantien prepared for fa jin. It is similar to the muscle tone that athletes maintain for quick response.

Most of us in our daily routines or exercises will at some point or another push our breathing to the maximum and at these points what is critical to us is acquiring enough air to sustain us. It is inspiration that concerns us, and we have little concern for expiration. This is because it is necessary to get quickly through with it so the next inspiration can occur. To maximize our breathing effectiveness, it is necessary to learn to control our expiration so that the maximum amount of air in our lungs is expired. Continual practice of this exercise will result in the adept more forcibly removing the air in his lungs and increase his capacity under duress. You should note that during fa jin the air is not forcibly removed, but instead a relaxed natural expulsion is desirable at the point of release.

1-12 The Tantien

The tantien is an energy center. It is the storehouse of qi. In martial applications the qi is stored in the tantien for immediate use. Without this storage of qi, there would be a time gap between the availability of produced qi and the martial need for the qi. The tantien is a midpoint location and is the locus of all forces entering and leaving the body. It is by focusing our attention on the tantien that we give it preeminence.

The tantien is located approximately two fingers below the navel, and approximately three fingers in from there. It can be more closely identified by panting much as an over heated dog does to dissipate heat. You can feel the tantien by placing you hand in that area as you pant.

Yi shou tantien, a common term within Taiji, literally translated means "mind's hand on the energy center." It means place your attention on the tantien. This removes the wisdom mind and its intent on action from the martial scene. Mind's hand on the tantien is an important factor in training the mental aspects of Taiji. It is by virtue of this centering of your attention on that point at or near the geometric center of mass that wei wu wei can occur. When you understand that much of the techniques of Taiji are devices that remove the wisdom mind from the application of techniques, then you will advance. Yi shou tantien's importance mainly lies within its ability to reduce the amount of intent involved in martial activity. In a sense, you are tricking the yi mind by carefully placing your attention on postures and other devices that keep the yi mind distracted and unable to force the movement. The movement must be allowed to happen and this can only occur if the yi mind steps aside.

1-13 Whole Body Power

The concept of whole body power is one of moving an accumulation of divergent energies amassed by manipulating the body as a coherent whole in a way that the forces are additive and result in constructive interference, rather than destructive interference. The term whole-body-power does not do it justice. It is a cluster of forces created by the interaction of mind body and spirit. This mind-body relationship is critical to understanding that po and the yi mind is at the center of it, and as we mature, there is a growing separation between the mental and physical aspects of our performance such that they destructively interfere with one another. Moving our body and mind in harmony to obtain a constructive effort so that each part contributes to the results is the basis of whole body power.

To accomplish whole body power requires reorganizing the way you think about power. If you perceive it as generated by li the musculature, then you will be limited to physical strength. It requires a leap of faith for most people to accept the fact that great power can be generated by very little muscular effort. It is this mental leap of faith that must first be trained in the candle method. With the first success at extinguishing the candle, comes that mental leap that must precede all physical efforts. It is a constant struggle to maintain this mental faith. It is easier to maintain this attitude during the expression of power than it is during the reception of power. Lazhu fangfa excels in this. If you understand that reception is the reverse of the expression of power, then you will know that each fa jin is also training in the reception of energy and the expression of energy as in whole body power. It is this multiple effect at the candle that accelerates the training of whole body power.

1-14 The Nature of Qi

While students are practicing fa jin before the candle, I quite often talk to them about the techniques they are attempting to utilize. I do this deliberately, not to instruct them, but rather to disengage the ego from the process. The ego can attend to only one thing at a time, and when it is engaged, po takes over control of bodily movement. This is how you can drive for miles and never know how you arrived at your destination. This quite often leads to an expression of surprise and glee on the part of the students, because without effort on their part, the qi flowed and extinguished the candle without their active intervention. There is a qualitative difference between the use of li and the unfettered expression of qi and you will feel that difference.

Without muscular tension, there is no kinesthetic feedback, so it is impossible to determine exactly what you have done. This lack of feedback is the most difficult aspect of the movement of qi, and when it is at its utmost, it is as if nothing happened. It is precisely this lack of feedback that makes qi so elusive. It works best without the ego intervention that is so predominant in most of the martial arts. Everything that facilitates the movement of qi is contrary to what a lifetime of effort states should be. Every strategy we have developed for success within the world must be thrown out and replaced with a new paradigm. The paradigm is that of the Taoist in which you do not use force against force, but instead move with the Tao so that you blend with nature and move in concert with it.

The storage of qi is within the muscular tension created by various postures, but the movement of the qi is by virtue of the relaxation of the same muscles. The qi follows the wave of relaxation created by successively relaxing muscles and flows to fill in this void left by the relaxation of muscles. The qi is stored locally within the muscular tension deliberately created for this purpose. This is the source of local qi, which so often accompanies the first attempt at any new physical endeavor. Quite often the first attempt at the candle is highly successful, and the following ones very frustrating. The student has exhausted the local qi and cannot duplicate the effort without knowing how to store and move qi

The Chinese use qi to define many things. It can mean the air that we breathe, energy, bio energy, etc. They have names for various types of energy. The qi they talk about is an energy that manifests itself in many ways. The qi released for fa jin is in many ways similar to pulse of energy released in a sine wave by the crack of a whip. The muscular effort or stored energy is released at the handle end by a thrust perpendicular to the length of the whip. This sends a sine wave pulse of energy throughout the length of the whip. There is a direct correlation between the amplitude of this sine wave and the frequency of the wave, as you decrease the amplitude of the wave there is an inverse relationship with the frequency, and it increases proportionally. The amplitude is depressed naturally in the whip by the rigidity of the material at the tip. The closer the wave gets to the end of the whip, the more rigid the material becomes, and this compresses the amplitude of the wave. This explains the jing, jin, or chin, depending on your spelling preference, that is mechanically produced by storage within the postures. This, however, is not the qi we seek. The qi that is important to us is that which is produced at the candle and results in an exclamation of surprise. It is that effortless result that seems to flow from nowhere, yet has surprising results. The exclamations of surprise are because we have not used muscles to produce this effect and consequently do not have any feedback to make us aware of the effort. The search for qi begins with the development of whole body power and ends with the elimination of all else but the ephemeral qi. It must be approached indirectly and the most effective way of training for it is with the candle method of Taiji called lazhu fangfa in Chinese. This method uses the candle flame as an indicator of the presence of qi. It is the staple of Yang style Taiji.

2

Principles of Mental Development

2-1 Theory of Sentient Consciousness

For internal martial purposes, the mind can be divided into three important aspects. These consist of the yi or wisdom mind, xin the heart mind (emotional mind) and po the ancient mind. The yi mind and xin mind are two separate aspects of hun, which is itself a part of hsing. Hsing is the essence of human nature; it is the yang side of this dichotomy and is the light, active principle. The yin side is ming. It is the life force, the dark, inactive principle and po is a part of it.

The external styles are more interested in the first two (yi and xin) and train in the latter by copying the characteristics of the ancient mind. It is the intention of the Taiji adept to utilize the yi mind in a direct effort to train the ancient mind with martial intent, so it can react to incoming energy and render it harmless at the direction of the yi mind.

Most styles utilize shasi qi (killing air) which is the attempt to intimidate the opponent by various means and render him ineffective. The kia of some styles and the grimace and external fear producing tactics are examples of shasi qi. Reserves of energy are created for immediate use and a formidable fighting style is released. This is not the manner of the internal styles. The weaknesses of the yi and xin minds must be understood. The use of an aggressive high energy emotionally charged attack strategy is a weakness of the external style martial art. These weaknesses will be discussed later. The difference between internal and external styles is in the particular strategy and the usage of the mental concepts in training, and there are additionally some fundamentally different means of generating power.

Within the mind of modern humans, there exist two parallel universes. On the one hand, we function in a world made up of words and social contexts, which are literally strung together by rational, linear thought. The second part of this universe is the world of geometric relationships, and patterns, one in which past and future are nonexistent. This is the eternal now. This is a geometric matrix created by this parallel existence of the ancient mind. The relationship between these two minds is reflected in the sinusoidal waves in which during the day the yi mind has preeminence and during sleep, the ancient mind has preeminence. The yi mind has invested a lifetime of effort in maintaining itself as the controlling, dominant one in this relationship, and it jealously guards this status with every device at its disposal.

The yi mind or wisdom mind is action oriented. It actively seeks to manipulate the environment for its own self-involvement. The yi mind has three aspects. They are desire, intensity of emotion and morality. Xin is the emotional aspect of the yi mind. It is that aspect of the mind that external styles cultivate for courage, resolve and intensity of effort based on aroused emotion. This is the shasi qi of the external styles, the "killing air." In self-preservation, quite often, the morality of the situation is often pushed aside in favor of a more pragmatic approach, and things are accelerated to an immediate maximum reaction. This immediate reaction to a threat is because of the emotional charge derived from the xin mind, which is trained to yield maximum effort. The ancient mind po is not imbued with desire, emotion or ego intent. It is in the realm of the reactive. It is reactionary in the sense that it responds to motion, brilliance, non-linear patterns and geometric shapes that have no correlation in the world of the yi mind. If you are working with intent, actively manipulating the environment for desired results, then you are within the domain of the wisdom mind (yi). The ancient mind works without benefit of kinesthetic feedback, without a moral compass and without fear. Fear is the domain of the ego. This fear inherent in the yi mind will cause it to withdraw from any situation unless the xin mind can override it. To train the ancient mind requires access to it. It is by way of this fear that we train po. In those situations where you are paralyzed by fear and cannot act, what has happened is that the yi mind has abdicated in favor of po. The ancient mind has no fear, so it is not fear that is paralyzing you. It is only that po is now preeminent. The importance lies in the fact that po does not fear death, but instead it has no concept of death. The concept of death requires the concepts of past and future, which are foreign to po. It is not that po does not fear death, it is that po lives in the "immediate and eternal now," and any concept beyond that is of no consequence. The ultimate finality of death is beyond its ability. Sequential thought is also beyond its ability. It thinks in terms of geometry and patterns of movement that may or may not be sequential in nature.

It is this fear reaction to a threat and the departure of the wisdom mind, and resultant emergence of po that interests us. We know that the yi mind and the ancient mind alternately trade preeminence and that it is with the yi mind that we are predominantly active. The paralysis that results in a threatening situation is not a true paralysis, but rather the emergence of the untrained po, that does not interpret the threat and does not react in a fearful way. The ancient mind does not move out of the way of a face smashing fist because it only "observes or monitors" the outer world and is concerned only with the inner workings of the body, but the important factor here is that it can be trained in specific ways to react in an acceptable martial way. There are specific ways in which po can be trained and the results can be awe-inspiring.

2-2 Cultivating the Warrior Mind

Considering the unique nature of the ancient mind, it is necessary to pattern the specific training methods in such a way as to address po and not the yi mind. This requires using techniques that will directly address po. To be able to train po, it is necessary first to be able to access it. Accessibility is something that is difficult, not by virtue of anything inherent in the nature of po, but because of the incessant demands of the wisdom mind for constant preeminence. It is in its nature to be always seeking constant affirmation as to its self-importance. It must be constantly told of its virtues and it seeks to thwart any effort to dislodge it from its seat of power.

The wisdom mind has a chink in its protection, which allows us to remove it from its preferred state of preeminence. There are three points of attack in which we can drive the wisdom mind from its dominance. We know that the wisdom mind craves constant feedback as to its superior qualities and constantly manipulates others to gain this reinforcement. What the wisdom mind is unable to tolerate is the boredom that is inherent in uninteresting non-feedback situations. Boredom is the natural enemy of this egomaniac. Ch'an (original Chinese version and precursor of Zen Buddhism of Japan) refers to this constant need for entertainment as the incessant chattering of a monkey leaping from tree to tree screaming at everything that moves. The mind is like this monkey.

Instead of leaping from tree to tree, it leaps from idea to idea constantly to reinforce its self-concepts as to its brilliance, beauty and social acumen. You hear much said of being able to still the mind, but it is not stillness of the wisdom mind we seek but rather the serenity of po. Stillness is not the goal, it is access to po and we accomplish this not by actively seeking stillness, because the active component is part of the wisdom mind. We seek it by driving the wisdom mind from preeminence by virtue of its incapability of tolerating boredom. We seek the escape from the wisdom mind by virtue of its greatest weakness, its incessant need for self-aggrandizement. Without this ego involvement, it is bored and it will retreat, and what is left is po. It is those moments of reverie with the departure of the ego functions that we get to know po. It is not direct knowledge, but we perceive it indirectly by the gaps in our attention, those periods of time in which we operate without being aware of what we are doing. It is a time of stillness. The chattering monkey has departed and the serenity of the moment although pleasing, is nevertheless unnoticed until the return of that incessant screaming idea manipulating tree climber reveals the contrasting nature between the two diverse states of mind when the internal dialogue once again returns.

Our strategy becomes one of occupying the wisdom mind with as many boring, repetitive and non self-serving activities as we can devise. The less rational or goal oriented it is the better. If it does not have any redeeming feature, what so ever, then it is so much the better. We must accost the wisdom mind on as many fronts as possible and we must do this for whatever length of time we can force our selves.

This then is our strategy, and if you remember anything, it is this concept that should always be foremost in your mind. The way to po is through the boredom of the wisdom mind.

The other two components of this triad we use to approach po besides boredom are fear and visualizations.

Fear has already been discussed. We will key in on that initial moment of aggression that creates this fear and the departure of the wisdom mind. This will be done in the training session. What is unique about visualizations is that they are different from imagination, which is an internal free play of ideas and imagery. This is a specific visualization without ideation, which is projected out into the environment, keyed to a perceived event, and sequenced properly so that when the event occurs, fear renders the wisdom mind inoperative, and po takes over, the technique to be employed is linked with the other components of the triad. It is a cluster of events which po will associate with the precipitating event. The repetitive nature of the practice will further serve to enhance the po aspect of the training.

2-3 The Form and the Warrior Mind

The form is practiced very slowly for many reasons. One reason is so that you can be self-correcting and make the needed corrections as they occur. Another reason is that it is difficult to maintain a position that is not properly balanced when moving in an exceptionally slow manner. It also requires you to pay close attention to posture and balance or encounter the strain and difficulty of sustained effort. There are many more reasons, but probably the most important is that the wisdom mind craves action. The slower you do the form, then the more boring it becomes. When you do it excruciatingly slow, then you can almost be assured that po is evident and you are doing the form, as it was intended.

The form is also done slowly so that we can practice the delicate transitions from one posture to another, and with correct foot and hand positions, which will reduce the time necessary for reaction. The postural preparatory positioning hands and the intermediate positions will greatly lower the reaction time. This is a distinct advantage when you are confronted by someone younger and faster than you are.

Many times, while doing the form, you will find yourself lost and you will not know where you are in the form. You have lapsed into po and the wisdom mind has escaped this boring interlude. This is good in the sense that in order for you to do the form, it is necessary that you force the wisdom mind to be in a situation it abhors. This constant interplay between the ancient mind and the wisdom mind is what we seek. It means that you are working on the interface of two opposing mindsets. This is exactly where we need to be. This struggle to escape the form means that any time it is necessary to apply the postures in a real situation, then, it is more likely that it will be po that is preeminent. You have in effect changed the normal sinusoidal conscious preeminence of the wisdom mind whenever it is associated with the form and therefore associated with conflict. This is to our advantage, and it means that when we do the form, it is po that we are training.

Remember boredom is your ally in this exercise. You are capitalizing on the weakness of the wisdom mind to train po. It is difficult to access po and train it, but in this instance what you do in the domain of the wisdom mind greatly influences po because of its close proximity with the yi mind.

If you are doing the form in the proper manner (mental frame of mind), then you will have difficulty in proceeding all the way through the form without some lapses of memory or having to stop and get your bearings as to where you are in the form. In the beginning stages, you are following, and this will not be a consideration. You must be aware, however, that this following represents the oscillation between yi and po and is a desirable condition when you finally begin to do the form on your own. It also assists in the development of following your opponent.

The concept of you xing zhie shi jia, wu xing fang wei zhen (having form is false, no form is the correct direction) uses these lapses of memory and it is something to be cultivated later when on a higher level your aim is to move into an area without form. It is not that you do not use the form as in practice; it is that you fight without the form.

2-4 Time Dilation and the Warrior Mind

Normal everyday processes have their own specific rate of temporal existence. Things move at a rate of speed to which we have become accustomed. It is our usual conception that this is the perceived rate in all situations, and that this must be a constant from person to person and from situation to situation. The rate at which we process information is dependent on how much processing must be done.

Time with respect to po or the ancient mind is reactive, based on a template we have devised through our training. This template is a shortened version of the one used by the wisdom mind. It is immediate and direct since past and future are not considerations of po, and fear is not possible as a disabling feature of the attack. Po does not operate in a social context, or utilize words, so information is not processed with regard to propriety or priority. This is the short list of possibilities, which can reduce the processing time.

It is not that time itself moves at a different rate, but that the processes within the mind of po have accelerated. Everyone else is operating at a level of time rate, which is much slower than po. It is as if all else was moving in slow motion. This is a perceived difference, which merely acknowledges the fact that you are operating in a mentally accelerated manner.

Most of us have experienced incidents within our own lives that lend credence to the existence of po and this otherworld existence. If you have been in a car wreck, you have experienced this apparent slowing down of time. Any experience, in which fear has transferred your awareness from the wisdom mind to po will illicit this temporal displacement.

For the martial artist, this has tremendous implications. If you can operate on a level that exceeds the youngest, fastest and most adept then you are at a distinct advantage. The truly amazing aspect of this is not that the physical attributes have given this advantage, but instead mental ones. This means that no matter how gifted or how hard the opponent trains, you have the advantage unless they too are operating within the realm of po.

2-5 The Cycle of Consciousness

We believe our daily existence to be constant and unchangeable, and we would be very much surprised to find how erratic and impermanent it is. We have seen others, and they have seen us when our eyes have glazed over and we have entered into some world unknown to us. Each day we move in and out of consciousness in a uniform and systematic way. The wisdom mind is dominant for the greater share of the cyclical wave of consciousness and po lurks in the periphery. It is the reverse at night. Quite often, what happens is that the wisdom mind in its incessant need to be pre-eminent will exhaust itself and during moments of boredom, we slip into a reverie in which time space and normal perception cease to exist. Many older societies use dancing to the point of exhaustion to access this nether world we call po. All societies have their means of access to the ancient mind that are unique to them, and they are predominantly using physical exhaustion as a means of causing the withdrawal of the wisdom mind. This is a total disruption of the normal cycle of consciousness. They usually select a time when the wisdom mind is most vulnerable, when the physical body is already beaten down from an exhausting day. This is a direct assault on the wisdom mind, and is not the method we use, even though the principles are the same. In a martial sense, we do not want to destroy the peak capability of the individual for the sake of acquiring po, but instead we must maintain our strength in the face of accessing po.

There is much that we do in training po that is similar to the techniques of sailing. To know where the wind is, sailors periodically luff the sails. This means that the boat is turned into the wind until the leading edge of the main sail flutters. This indicates that you have headed too far into the wind and you have lost the effectiveness of the sail. If you move away from the wind too far, then you stall the boat in the same manner as an airplane is stalled when the angle of attack is too great, but there is no perception of this. Other than the slowing of the boat, which can be almost imperceptible, there is no indication that you have fallen off from the wind and are stalling the boat. Luffing then allows you to measure where the wind is and to assure you that the boat is not in a stall.

This dance between the wisdom mind and po is much like this scalloping motion that periodically occurs in sailing. We are intent on walking that fine line between po and the wisdom mind. There are devices for traversing this no man's land, and they will be explained later. For now, just remember that there is a fine line we must traverse and everything we do is centered on keeping po and the wisdom mind in close proximity.

2-6 Yin and Yang

Yin and yang have been given so much coverage that it is not necessary to delve into it as most literature deals with it adequately. It is important to make distinctions with respect to this fine line we are traversing between the wisdom mind and po. Po can be correlated with the soft slow aspects of Taiji and the wisdom mind with those active, hard forceful activities that compose the external styles. It is by no accident that the internal styles typically emphasize the soft aspect of martial intervention. Just as with the physical aspects of yin and yang, those mental aspects are also reflected in the yin and yang cycle of activity. There is a yin and yang interplay of forces within the form. It is soft by design, but its complexity requires the attention of the wisdom mind because without it we lapse into reverie with no martial gain. The smooth flow of energy during the form increases the probability of these lapses and if we are doing the form properly, they will occur. It is the yang portion of this sinusoidal wave that yanks us back to the form and we continue. It is by virtue of these episodes of yin and yang that we know that we are traversing that thin line and that both the wisdom mind and po are attending to the training, much as luffing the sail indicates how close to the wind we are.

2-7 The Temple Guard

In training, it is imperative that we search for the temple guard. This is the guardian or egocentric part of the personality that maintains preeminence of the wisdom mind. When we find the temple guard, then we know that our training has been effective. We search by keeping uppermost in our minds the realization that the closer we are to po then the crazier the temple guard becomes.

The chattering monkey, which is the temple guard, is susceptible to enticement, and a trap can be set. The Hindus have a means of capturing the monkey. It is called a monkey trap and consists of a glass milk bottle with a rope tied to it. This is then tied to a tree and an orange is placed within the bottle, and it is highly visible to the monkey. This is an irresistible presentation and the monkey will without fail reach for the orange. He will find that he cannot remove the orange with it held in his hand. The monkey does not make the connection between "letting go," and acquiring the desired object.

Most of us have monkey traps in our lives. They consist of those things of which we cannot let go, even when they prevent us from acquiring that which we desire most. For martial purposes, this temple guard signals for us that something we are doing is a threat to the preeminence of the wisdom mind. The truth is that when we feel that we have failed; then the incessant chattering of the monkey (temple dog) is in essence what is preventing us from doing what we desire and all we have to do is let go of the orange. By intervening in the process with the wisdom mind, we prevent our accomplishments from coming to fruition.

By understanding the devices of the wisdom mind and training ourselves to deceive the temple guard and by letting go of our need to control every situation, then we can then travel this fine line between the two opposing worlds. We do this by veering into the wind and backing off from the wind to maintain the optimum configuration as in sailing. On the po, side is the loss of the effort in the form, the trance-like loss of awareness in performing the form, and on the other side is the internal dialogue that also stops our concentration and attention in performing the form. It requires a balancing act in which the mind is stilled to stop the incessant chatter, and additionally the mind is maintained in a non-controlling but aware manner such that the form can be performed. Without this attention, we even forget to perform the next part of the form.

2-8 Wu Wei

Wu wei is a process. It is in a sense, doing without doing. The concept is found within the I Ching by Lao Tzu. It occurs there in the form wei wu wei. Wu wei actually means non-action. The proper term is wei wu wei, which means action by means of non-action. It is also called the empty mind or no-mind. I say it is a process because it is action without the intervention of the wisdom mind. This is a concept that is zhen qi guai or very strange, which is little understood, and talked about in hushed tones, referenced yet undefined, and usually it is not directly addressed. It is in reality the process of performing some action while in the state of po. Wu wei is the activity, and po is the inactive state of being. Thus the term wu wo (not me) is derived. It is something other than me that is performing.

Zen archery is a perfect example. The bow is drawn and the mind is stilled until "it moves me" and the arrow flies. The (it) that moves you is po. Wu wei is the act of waiting until you have accessed po, and then allowing the mysterious po to operate without interference from the yi or wisdom mind. Because there is a lack of feedback from po, it has the appearance of action by inaction. Not doing is the act of utilizing the processes of po accompanied by the feeling of the absence of active attempt on your part due to this lack of feedback. The highly popularized paradox of wei wu wei, action without action is a product of the yi mind. It is by virtue of imposing a logic and its imperative premise on a given situation that we arrive at the paradox of wu wei. It is our concept of cause and effect that is violated because the lack of feedback does not allow us to pinpoint the source or cause of the action.

The martial arts are a way of life in which we discipline our center of attention in a specific way. We attend to things that in our ordinary, everyday life are ignored. In the form, the tantien is an insertion point for our attention. We actively move from this central point. We also visualize the opponent and his relationship to the posture of the moment and thus train ourselves visually in the proper recognition of techniques. Stilling the mind also is a technique utilized to access po. It works because we use the intense focus of our attention on some aspect of the environment (the tip of our nose for instance) to either fatigue the yi mind or bore it so that it escapes the situation. It is this deliberate intervention in the activity of the yi mind and the restriction of it that encompasses all of the techniques of stilling the mind.

2-9 The Periphery of Perception

The visual field is typically divided into two separate areas of function. The center or fovea is primarily concerned with visual acuity and color vision, and the rods and cones are at a higher concentration. The periphery of vision is predominantly made of rods and is concerned with movement. Color is decreasingly evident in the peripheral areas. These distinctions are relevant to the external and the internal styles. Within the external styles, the fovea or the focused visual field of the eye is the domain of the wisdom mind.

The internal styles, in order to function in a soft and yielding manner, must operate within the domain of po so that the dilation of time is emergent and mental action is accelerated. The domain of po is on the periphery of vision, and not only will you stop the flowing movement of your body, if you are focused on the ten thousand things in the center of vision, but you will also prevent yourself from entering po. This will stop the natural flow of your mind because you will become fixated on whatever is in the center of the visual field.

The peripheral vision is an area where color vision is absent, clear focused vision is in the fovea and absent in the periphery. Motion and spatial orientation are predominant in the periphery. This is the domain of po. This combination of spatial orientation and motion coupled with the time dilation evident in po is the martial arena within which the internal styles operate. It is not the wisdom mind, but we do tend to operate in that in-between state, which borders on and cycles between the two as the situation demands.

The time dilation, precise spatial coordination and motion detection are fundamental to a soft yielding type interception that renders the opponent vulnerable. It is this acceleration of thought processes that make this interception workable. One of the important sayings within Taiji is that "he does not move, I do not move, if he moves, I move first." This can only be done by accessing po and keying in on specific points of the opponents attack. If he starts first, then the only way we can arrive first is by this acceleration of mental process combined with a triggering means.

If your attention is focused on the periphery then your mind is attending to only those aspects of the surrounding environment that involve moving energy and the intent to use it against you. Force has been relegated to incoming and outgoing energy as a moving object that only needs to be tracked and intercepted. The response is immediate and effective if trained properly.

3

Mental Prowess

3-1 Theory of Mental Imagery

Imagery is the necessary by product of a mind that does not use words. It is this manipulation of patterns of imagery and geometric designs that comprise the ancient mind. Words are a relatively new innovation in the evolution of thought over the millennium mammalian life has existed, and it occurs in the more recent developments of the human mind. They are not a part of the ancient mind. If we still the mind, we eliminate words; therefore, the only way to manipulate thought within the domain of po is through imagery. Without words to assert its preeminence, the wisdom mind recedes into a daydream state that is resplendent with mental imagery. We dream of great accomplishments, picturing them with relish in a fantasy world that has a reality of its own, until shattered by a word, any word. As long as we can maintain this stillness of mind, we can operate within this sphere. The stillness must come from this relaxed sentience and not be forcefully and intentionally accomplished by the wisdom mind. It is by virtue of the wisdom mind stepping aside and allowing this to happen, that this state occurs.

We can manipulate the wisdom mind by manipulating words, and it will hover around and be avidly interested in all intimations that it is important. Po also is susceptible to manipulations. These however, must be in the form of visual images. In both instances, we are manipulating the perception of reality. We can also manipulate po by setting up desired intention. We can do this by constant repetition and intensifying the effort with concomitant induced emotional content. This must be done without words, and with intense vivid visualizations. You become good at this by practice, as with everything else, the more you do it the better you are at it.

It must be noted, that po is not the right side of the bicameral brain, a popular conceptualization today. This deals with the phenomenal world, the ten thousand things. Po has another separate world of existence. It deals with energy relationships and is buried deep within the primitive recesses of the reptilian mind.

The wisdom mind also deals with visualizations and symbolic thought much as po does. It is through this means that the two can communicate. It is by raising the level of emotional intensity that the wisdom mind can convey its intents and desires to po through mental imagery. This emotional intensity is determined by po to be an increase in energy level. It then becomes an imperative.

3-2 Visualizations and their Usage

Visualizations are in the arena of the wisdom mind, and imagery is in the domain of po. The distinction between the two other than semantics is that with the wisdom mind visualization is based on intent, an active intervention, or deliberate fabrication of a visual image. Within po, the imagery is the product of a separate but equally true alternative reality and it is not actively manipulated in any manner. The visualization is the same as reality. It is important to repeat this for emphasis. The visualization for po is the same as reality irrespective of the actual conditions that exist.

Visualizations serve our martial purpose because it is a means of access to po. We can manipulate the visualization with enough intensity of effort within the domain of the wisdom mind, and with enough emotion to convince po that this is reality and then po will act accordingly. The truly effective aspect of visualizations is the fact that you actually do not have to perform whatever technique you are studying but can use visualizations to perfect the sequence. Of course, actual practice helps, but great gains can be made with predominantly visual techniques. These gains can be accomplished only if you in fact are actually accessing po.

It is possible to accomplish hundreds of times more practice sessions without actually doing them and without the fatigue, which serves as a limiting factor. As you do the form, you should be keeping the sense of the opponent before you at all times. This is a visualization technique that uses this access to po to train you in applying the technique to a given situation. If you know where the opponent is then your reaction is appropriate to a real situation. These visualizations should also be accompanied by creating the appropriate memories of the kinesthetic sensations that accompany the actual techniques.

3-3 Static Imagery and its Effect

Just as we can use words to affect the behavior of the wisdom mind, so too can we use static imagery to affect the behavior of po. Various forms of static imagery such as the stylized renderings of the chakras can yield effects in meditation, and more readily advance you into desired alternate states. These are readily used in some yogic traditions, and tumo of the Tibetan monks. The Tibetans use a stylized version of the sun to implement their techniques. These techniques work because they mimic actual alternate reality conditions or images.

The Chinese language grew out of stylized pictographs of meaningful symbolism in the distant past. The colorful descriptive names that the ancient warriors gave their techniques had meaningful messages in them that enhanced their instructive value for the student. Much of this cultural color is lost to the western practitioner.

This imagery is called static to differentiate it from the on going active imagery that is part of our daily mental life. It is static in the sense that in comparing it, for instance, to the actual chakras, it is a fixed picture, while the chakras themselves are moving processes that is very complicated sequence of events. They work, not because they are duplication of the event itself, but rather as a triggering device, which can precipitate the event, and used as such they can be quite effective.

Static images in the martial sense are abundant in the Shaolin (xiaolin) community. Temples are resplendent with imagery and examples of techniques and important concepts. Every posture within the form is a snapshot or picture that is symbolic of a technique that is much more complicated that the actual posture. The form is a symbolic representation of each technique and the form transitions smoothly from one to the other in a flowing manner.

3-4 Pedagogic Imagery

Imagery works primarily because it is non-verbal. Its usage as a training device is based on the fact that it is a non-verbal method of accessing po. We could give a verbal dissertation all day long and po would not be impressed or even understand it. The form as it is presented in pictures is a form of pedagogic imagery. Key points in the form are depicted so that you have guideposts to lead you from one technique to the other. Chinese culture and especially the Xiaolin temples have wall drawings depicting various postures. Everything that occurs within the training cycle is done with a progression from words to images. The ancients used words that led to very descriptive images, which can evoke a response from po.

One prime example of this is the term beautiful lady's hand which immediately elicits the image of a graceful arcing hand and forearm that is connected, smooth and delicate, one that moves as a connected whole in a delicate manner, yet contains great strength and resolve. This is a means of bridging that gap between the world of words of the wisdom mind and the world of imagery of po. The martial world of the Buddhist and Taoist is replete with this type of pedagogic imagery.

The term beautiful, lady's hand has a cluster of images that are associated with it for specific training purposes. The graceful arc is reminiscent of the circular movements that are characteristic of Taiji. The graceful transition of the arm through the wrist to the hand creates smooth transition for the qi and prevents the whipping of the hand at the wrist, which will cause the harmful focus of all energy at that point. The gracefulness of a beautiful woman elicits imagery of the softness and gentleness that is inherent in the Taoist philosophy. Another term for the beautiful lady's hand is yu nu shou. This is jade lady's hand. Even though we are not of that culture, it conjures up imagery of delicate finery and the beautiful lady.

It is through this transition from words to images that po is trained. It is in the form of all of those colorful descriptions of the stances, which are designed to elicit specific images that we explore the mysterious world of po.

There is another more potent form of training with visualizations that is more effective in a martial point of view. This comprises using sequence visualizations such as interception and attack sequences. These work because even if we lie down and do not move at all, there are minute muscular movements that accompany each thought. The direction arrow for learning is from the muscular to the mental. What this means is that we first learn by doing and then apply words and logic to it afterwards. A good example of this is the learning of the name for the letter "A." We spend considerable time writing the letter "A." Even before we practice it, there are eye movements that trace the symbol in its entirety, and these eye movements are memorized. Everything we visualize is a memorization of earlier visualized muscular memories. If we visually see the letter "A," then we make these minute muscular eye and hand movements that depict the letter "A."

What we do in visualizations, within the martial arena, is reverse this process. We visualize the particular activity in which we are interested and then the muscular sensations and minute movements that characterize it will occur in conjunction with the visualization. All the same, movements, calculations, and geometric relationships with the visualization occur as it would if it were happening in real time. It is therefore possible to gain the exact same effect with visualizations as it is with actual practice. This is important in Taiji because it is the softness and skill level of the technique we are interested in, and not the muscular benefit.

3-5 Fear of Heights and Imminent Danger

Part of the built in circuitry within the human mind is the fear of heights above ten feet. As we ascend in height, we become increasingly apprehensive. The functioning of our binocular vision serves not only to tell us distance off of a target, but it also serves to warn us of impending danger due to possible fall from a height. This built in warning system functions to warn us of the potential threat. It is the wisdom mind that is preeminent in this warning system. As we stated earlier, po has no fear and does not comprehend beyond the immediate eternal now. This distinction between the fear of heights and the lack of this fear will serve as a means of differentiating between our presences in either of these states. If fear is prevalent in our present state of being, then we exist within the realm of the wisdom mind and not po. We can capitalize on this distinction for training purposes.

3-6 The Edge of the Precipice

Infants while in the crawling stage exhibit a strange behavior. When they cross a barrier, which can be represented by a pattern change such as a paint line on the floor, they will stop. It is not a function of binocular vision, but one of discrimination between an existing pattern and the change to a new pattern. A simple black line on the floor will elicit this response in a baby. The recognition of patterns is a function of the imagery of the ancient mind.

We see this as it occurs in adults by that unreasonable fear we experience as the edge of a building is approached, a ledge or some other demarcation point at a height. It is not the height we fear but the demarcation. In rappelling off the top of a cliff, there is an initial fright that must be overcome, and once we are on the face of the cliff, then we are no longer fearful. This is because the demarcation point has disappeared and the edge with it.

This is another point of distinction between existence in the wisdom mind and the non-fearful existence in po. The distinction here is that po does not exhibit any fear, but the response is merely one of stopping the behavior. The response in the wisdom mind is one of fear, an emotional response that makes one tentative in the presence of the feared object. It is this distinction that tells us if we are within the domain of po or not.

3-7 Nocturnal Flying

Some of us dream of flying, but most of us do not. Flying in a dream exceeds the bounds of the rational mind. The wisdom mind cannot comprehend doing the impossible, even in a dream. What is even worse is deliberately placing oneself at risk by exceeding that limit of ten feet and positioning oneself on the edge of a precipice to launch oneself into the dreamscape is more than the wisdom mind can fathom. It is predisposed to escape when it is threatened. If you launch yourself within a dream from that edge which your senses tell you will be certain death and you succeed, then your state of being is po. The wisdom mind cannot place itself into such a terrifying situation. Therefore, po will be pre-eminent. It is by deliberately dreaming of flying that one can train in accessing po.

3-8 Dreaming

The dream world can be characterized by some distinct phases that one goes through to access deep sleep. One of the first stages we go through on the way to deep sleep is what is now called REM sleep. This is an acronym for Rapid Eye Movement. This is easily picked up on an electroencephalogram (brain wave pattern). This characterizes entry into that hypnotic state between wakefulness and deep sleep. In this state, we are dreaming and we cycle in and out of this state approximately every ninety minutes. During this state, the brain waves indicated by an electroencephalogram would indicate a state close to wakefulness. Each state from deep sleep to alert wakefulness is delineated by a consistent frequency pattern, which for didactic purposes has been separated into four stages. These are deep sleep with a frequency range of delta .5-3.5 cycles per second, theta from 4-7 cycles per second, alpha from 8-13, and total wakefulness in math or problem solving beta waves from 14-30 cycles per second.

The importance of this cyclical behavior of the REM. state is that we know it is approaching wakefulness and we need to know in what state we are. It is important that we cycle our consciousness in close to the wisdom mind such that we can slip back into po with little effort. The problem is that it is important for us to know in which state of mind we are at this particular moment. How you can make this distinction between po and the yi mind and how to utilize dreaming is an important part of training.

From earlier discussion, we know that the edge has some relevance for us. It is apparent that if you stand on the edge of great height that the wisdom mind, fearing the consequences of your actions, is preparing to flee the situation. The wisdom mind is not going to allow you to do this irrational thing. As you stand on the edge of the precipice in your dream, visualize yourself leaping in a swan dive and then soaring to great heights. If you can accomplish this, it is po that is preeminent. It should be evident that not only can you talk to po through colorful imagery in the description of stances, but that you can also access po through dreaming and set up tasks to be trained in the dream state. It is important to note that the closeness of po and the yi mind is evident in the fact that you dreamed of vivid flying and that you remembered it. If you were only within po then you would not have remembered it, as with most dreams.

The preoccupation of the Chinese martial arts with flying and great leaps in their movies probably has its origin in this type of qi gong and martial arts training.

3-9 Training Effects of Imagery

Training the mind with visualization and keying these directly to performance in the form or fight sequence practice at the candle (Lazhu Fangfa) is probably more effective than regular training. This is true because you are training that aspect of the mind which deals directly with the perceived environment and its responses are immediate and direct. The wisdom mind is encumbered by all the social contexts prevalent in the situation. It must select the proper moral and ethical standard to be applied to the situation. The wisdom mind is very easily intimidated in most of us. It will escape the immediate threat and leave an untrained po to handle the situation. This untrained aspect of the mind will stand there without fear and calmly watch as a high velocity fist approaches. Many of us have been in this situation, and have since trained ourselves accordingly. It is, however, not the same training as we are talking about here.

Conventional training accesses the wisdom mind and trains at the center of focus of the eye. It can be quite good, and unquestionably fast, but what is missing is that particular attack which comes from the side, which is out the center of the visual field. Seldom does an attack come from the front with warning, posturing, and all the accouterments of the movie scenario. The Marquis of Queensberry rules do not apply here. The opponent will take every advantage and leave you none.

The specifics of training will be given later, what is important here is that you get an understanding of the merits of training the ancient mind. It is a difficult concept to get across. It is not something that can be readily displayed to show your skills. Much of the training you do is based on your faith that in an actual situation you will perform as you have trained. Most of our experience is to the contrary of our training method. This is why internal styles are so difficult to learn. Much of what passes as internal training is merely a soft version of the external styles. To train internally, you must train the ancient mind.

3-10 Kinesthetic Imagery

Up to this point, all that has been discussed is visual imagery. One very important aspect of training is the kinesthetic sensations that accompany all training. By paying attention to those kinesthetic sensations that occur during training and by attempting to reproduce them in the mental visualization of the technique, you can enhance your training. This occurs because even though you are just visualizing the technique, there are corresponding muscular contractions, although minor, they serve to train muscle memory. By duplicating kinesthetic sensations, we pinpoint the training more specifically to just those muscles involved in the performance. We assure ourselves of the proper placement of the hand foot etc. by reinforcing the proper kinesthetic memory.

3-11 The Imagery of Chan Sichou

The term chan sichou is derived from the ancient silk culture of China. Chan sichou literally means "silk reeling." When the slender thread is pulled from the silk worm's cocoon, it causes the cocoon to spin and rotate in the spiral pattern (figure eight) that the silk worm used in placing it on the cocoon. The silk worm anchors itself at the posterior end and by rotating from this one point; it creates a spiral pattern that completely encloses it, except for a small opening at the top. This opening is the last point sealed and it closes in the cocoon. This spiraling pattern is the imagery of chan sichou. As we move from posture to posture, we are storing this spiraling energy in the musculature of the body. Every turning point or twist of the torso in the form is an opportunity to store energy.

With the utilization of chan sichou, the kinesthetic imagery is of great importance. It is with kinesthetic imagery that chan sichou is perfected. If you do not feel these sensations, then you are not performing it properly. Your foot is then improperly placed or your balance is not on the proper leg. You can mentally rehearse these sensations along with the visualizations and perfect your technique.

Chan sichou is one of the important ways in which we store energy in the body. The rotation of the body over a planted foot and this twist of the musculature, which is reminiscent of a child on a swing that is twisted in a spiral and then let free, and the stored energy when released then spirals back to the original position. It is this release, which is of importance. The energy must be allowed to return by releasing it and allow it to freely flow back to its original position. If you actively try to force it back into position, you are using the musculature of the body to move the arm etc. and in doing so; you are avoiding the effect of song.

3-12 Nine Pearls

The nine pearls are essentially the joints. First in the sequence of the pearls as they are positioned from the rear, grounded foot to the tips of the finger is the yongquan point located on middle of the ball of the foot. From the foot to the finger tips the sequence is the yongquan point; the ankle (jiaowan); the knee (xi); the hip (tunbu); the sacrum; the ming men; the shoulder (jianbang); the elbow (zhou) and finally the wrist (shouwan).

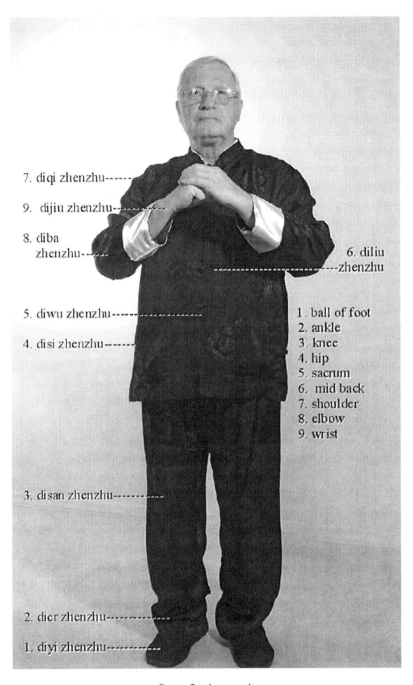

7. diqi zhenzhu-----
9. dijiu zhenzhu-------
8. diba zhenzhu------
6. diliu zhenzhu-------
5. diwu zhenzhu-----
4. disi zhenzhu------
3. disan zhenzhu----------
2. dier zhenzhu-----------
1. diyi zhenzhu-----------

1. ball of foot
2. ankle
3. knee
4. hip
5. sacrum
6. mid back
7. shoulder
8. elbow
9. wrist

figure 3. nine pearls

In the martial arena, these connections serve as a flow line of jing as it is transported from the compression and torque of the yongquan through each connection to the fingertips. These connections must be proper or the jing produced will be dissipated in any defective pearl. The imagery here is that of a pearl held in place in a specific location by a knot as seen in a string of pearls. They are strung in the sequence taken by the lines of force generated by the jing begun at the grounded foot. These connections allow the transmission of the energy across what normally would be loosely connected joints and delivers it to the release point, and careful attention to these connections must be taken to elicit the proper connection. This must be done without creating a muscular tension along the route, otherwise at the moment of relaxation and flow of qi there would be a constriction to the smooth flow of qi. When the classics say to extend the qi, it means that you must make these connections so that there can be a free flow of qi. These joint connections are a primary method of delivering force through the body. Constant reminders of the nine pearls and the imagery of each pearl strung together to form a complete necklace, is sufficient for most of us to maintain this continuity. Remember that severing the string of pearls will send them all in a cascade to spill on the ground. As we progress, we will change from viewing this as a necklace of important points to one of an image of a continuous meridian for the flow of energy.

3-13 The Nine Bends in the Pearl

Instead of a path drilled through the pearl to allow it to be strung, this imagery is that of a convoluted passage with nine bends. This imagery invokes the difficulty of threading the pearl through these convolutions. In order to move through this difficult path of nine pearls, you must place the yi mind on each pearl to thread the qi through this channel in the proper sequence. It is possible to force the jing through these nine pearls and the nine bends in the pearl, but the qi will not flow at all unless these connections are perfect. Much of the training in Taiji is to establish this difficult passage, so that you may place the qi anywhere in the body that you choose. The nine bends are a visualization technique that keeps the awareness of the difficult passage uppermost in your thoughts.

3-14 Imagery as a Mnemonic Device

The methods and practices of the martial arts were derived in a culture that was predominantly illiterate. To assist those in training, memory devices were employed to facilitate the learning process. Many of these devices were derived from the imagery and symbolism of the existing culture. The exact meaning of much of this is lost even to those currently a part of the Chinese culture. Meanings and symbolism change with the progression of years, and the new meanings may not reflect the original intent. It then becomes a matter of determining what works and what does not to rectify this disparity. The true nature of the knowledge that existed at that time is not what has been handed down. We have only the training methodology and little of the thoughts of the intellectuals of the time.

The Chinese language presents its own problems. Most of the written characters have immense symbolism associated with their meanings. Some of this symbolism and imagery is obvious, but much is lost in antiquity.

4

Qi and Its Applications

4-1 Definition of QI

Within the Chinese language, qi has many meanings. It can mean air; there is prenatal qi; post natal qi; the original essence qi; the energy of qi that flows through the meridians etc. The list is long and varied. The martial definition of qi is that of a force which is directed through the body by the wisdom mind and delivered to the hand, foot etc. which results in a disruption of the flow of qi in the opponent. Jing is the kinetic equivalent of the force produced by the manipulation of muscles, tendons, fascia, body postures etc., that yield a pulsed force that can be delivered to the hand foot etc.

The difference is that qi occurs, seemingly without the intervention of the musculature, which is evident in the transmission of jing. It is the absence of muscular effort that characterizes the effects of qi. This is why song is so important in the early training in Taiji. It is by learning to move the body with very little musculature and being connected at the nine pearls that qi is able to flow. In storing the qi, we collect it in various parts of the body by muscular contraction and torsion, then release the tension, and allow the stored qi to flow as directed by the wisdom mind. The direction of the flow of qi by the wisdom mind is complicated and will be dealt with later, but for now, it is sufficient to think of qi as filling the vacuum left by the relaxation of the muscles. With jing, you actively, mentally and physically, manipulate the body in order to produce force. The manipulation of qi initially produces a force that results from the reduction in usage of muscles, and the effort at manipulation of the body. It is by gradually reducing the muscular effort that we begin to see the results of the manipulation of qi

4-2 Theory of Qi

Qi is an intrinsic energy and as such, it moves through the body to supply the energy source for various ongoing functions of the body to sustain it as a viable living entity. To understand qi, it is necessary to familiarize yourself with the relationship of the various aspects of existence. This begins with the concept, which is referred to as the "vast unknown." It is a state of wu qi or an undifferentiated existence. The first separation or movement within wu qi is Taiji and it is then separated into yin and yang. Picture the tao diagram listed previously with a column on the left, which is the yang side, and a column on the right, which is the yin portion. The yang portion represents the body. It should be noted that po, which can be defined as spirit, moves its point of observation within this separation. The yang aspect of human existence is then separated into hun, which is the physical existence, the world of yiwan dongxi or the ten thousand things, which is all that we can comprehend as existing. Qi is manipulated throughout the body and it is used to manipulate the body in the sense of the classical concepts of deus ex machina, the ghost within the machine. The physical body does indeed seem as if it is designed with a set of trip levers that could be operated by a ghost or soul and made to function in a mechanical way. It is po, which manipulates the body. Hun (yi mind aspect) in close cooperation with po directs the nature of the movement of the body. The closer in tune with each other that po and hun are, then this relationship operates in an efficient and mutually beneficial way. It is when hun interferes in an effort to capture control for its own gratification difficulties will arise. Because qi is manipulated and delivered by po, difficulties can occur in the direct manipulation and the understanding of qi. Because qi is only manipulated by po, it is therefore necessary to understand this relationship between hun and po to gain some insight into the nature of qi and its manipulation. Preeminence within this dual relationship is excessively valued by hun. It is important to note that hun lives within the mind and po lives within the body. For all its simplicity and lack of sophistication, it is po that is the more complex. It sits in the unique position of being able to look in both directions. It can access the phenomenal world, the world of the ten thousand things, and the Tao. How this can happen requires some explanation of this relationship between po and hun.

There are three different and separate forms of existence to which we as humans are exposed. These are shen, hun and po. There is an identity, an observer that moves within each state of being which is no more than a nugget of awareness that assumes these different and disparate forms of existence to manipulate the environment within each of them. This is shen. The nature of this existence will be discussed in Section Four of this book. It should be noted that the observer oscillates from one to the other and does not reside in more than one at a time. It only appears that it does when it rapidly oscillates.

This relationship is discussed so that the nature of qi and its relationship to existence can be identified. Psychokinesis has been statistically established by the J. B. Rhine studies. It has been established by reputable scientists with such precision that if you cannot accept the findings within that study, then you must throw out all sub atomic physics and any other science that utilizes statistical methods. To confound the issue further, the problem of action at a distance and the lack of attenuation over distance add further fuel to the fire. However, science has other instances of this and their devices to smooth it out are many. Gravity is a similar problem, in that action at a distance is difficult to resolve. This is resolved by field theory, which explains nothing, but is a device to circumvent the problems. Gravity has another problem, and it is that in order to have the mathematics match the reality, the calculations, for instance in orbital decay, must postulate the instantaneous interaction of forces between the two objects, in total violation of the speed of light limit. It is also interesting that telepathy also has this unique problem, and does not seem to have the time delay required over long distances and it is not attenuated by these distances. The low level of performance in these studies just might be attributable to access to po.

Because the exact nature of qi is not known, and it is on the fringes of measurement capability, it is necessary to talk around it. Like the iron filings in a magnetic field, we can talk about its effects, even if we do not know its exact nature.

We can say with certainty that it operates instantaneously at a distance the same way gravity does, and that the strength of the signal is not attenuated by the square of the distance. We can also say that it moves throughout the body according to Taoist tradition, through a meridian system and that this flow can be manipulated by po. For martial purposes, it is not the meridian flow that is manipulated, but instead, it is the flow through the tissues other than at the meridians. The hun aspect can manipulate this energy by virtue of its relationship with po. It is this observer or immortal of the Chinese that oscillates between the two states of being on an everyday basis. The movement of this observer to the po aspect is a more tenuous arrangement, since it is also a state of being and the real existence is the observer, or immortal zhen zheng ren.

Qi is instrumental in the psychokinetic and telepathic natures of man. It is through qi that both of these occur. The nature of qi is such that it can heal or destroy. This determination is a function of the application not the energy itself. Telepathy is firmly embedded in the evolutionary aspects of man. It is by virtue of this relationship between po and hun that difficulties arise with its usage. This difficulty is of the nature of access and signal strength. It is directly accessible through po and depending on signal strength, is accessible through hun. The difficulty of accessing it through po is that it is nonverbal and not always easily understood on the hun level. Psychokinesis as with telepathy is accessible through po and indirectly through hun. Both of these paranormal abilities are manifestations of the use of qi, and like the iron filings in a magnetic field, they allude to the fact of the presence of qi. Its usage within martial arts is in the area of ting jing (sensing power) and fa jin (striking power). In both instances, it is qi that is being utilized in various degrees. It is just the manner in which it is utilized that is different.

4-3 Cultivating the Movement of Qi

Determining the actual movement of qi is difficult, because its movement is at the discretion of po. Within the realm of po, there is no bodily feedback of kinesthetic, motor proprioceptors, or other sensory information. Feed back occurs within the wisdom mind aspect of hun, and it then becomes necessary to utilize the feedback system of information within the realm of hun and create situations in which the movement of qi can occur and utilize the feed back of some accompanying activity that has feedback to tie the two together.

It has been known early on by the Taoist that muscular activity results in the movement of qi to the area of activity. This is one of the basic tenets of qi gong. Qi gong is a precursor to much of the knowledge of the energy system within the body. It predates the martial arts, and the oldest records of activities in this area refer to breathing through the heels, which is a direct reference to qi gong. This is the movement of qi from the ground through the body in coordination with breathing. A person that breathes through his heels is considered an immortal or "true human," zhenzheng ren, an enlightened individual, a sage person.

Even though our goal is to eliminate muscular effort, we can use this method of accumulating qi and use the kinesthetic sensations as a guide to the movement of qi, and at the same time eliminate the muscular tension at appropriate times. We can then have the accumulation of qi through muscular effort and the relaxation of muscular tension with the accompanying sensations of the movement of qi. We can use this as a training tool. As a preliminary to the actual control of qi, this allows us to work within the area of hun, which we can control, and access qi without the complicated mechanisms required when accessing po. We will train this access to po at a later date.

We will use the attempt to store qi by muscular effort to create sensations that we can identify in association with this effort, and then we can relax the muscles in a controlled manner such that a wave of relaxation of the muscles results in a kinesthetic sensation of the movement of this wave and this sensation can be associated with the movement of qi. This wave of relaxation results in the flow of qi into the vacuum of tension left behind by this wave of relaxation. These are sensations that we can cultivate, and we can use this wave of muscular relaxation to train the movement of qi. This is the beginning stage of training the movement of qi. Later, the training of the movement of qi can be moved to the realm of po.

There are specific training methods that can be used to train the movement of qi within the realm of hun. Much of the training within qigong is of this nature.

4-4 The Energy System of the Body

The normal circulation of energy within the body is the fire path. This consists of the movement of qi down the ren mei or conception vessel at the front of the body and up the governing vessel or du mei at the back. This normal path of circulation is what is used for external martial purposes. It is for enlightenment purposes that the energy is led through the "back flowing" process that is the reverse direction. This is the water path, and the flow is upward in front on the ren mei and downward on the du mei or back. The Taoist tradition considers this "backward flowing" process essential to Chin Hua the "Golden Flower" or enlightenment.

Within the fire path the ren mei or Conception Vessel, qi flows down until it meets the hui yin at the base of the torso, which is considered a restriction to the flow of qi, from there it flows upward within the du mei or governing vessel.

The back or du mei is considered yang or positive while the front of ren mei is considered yin in nature. Taiji uses the yang upward flowing energy system at the du mei (Fire Path) for fa jin (the striking arts) in the ming jing and an jing levels of force and the yin downward flowing energy system at the du mei for the soft jings and hua jing. It is this "backward flowing" process within the energy system that has given rise to the idea that Taiji is a walking meditation. This "backward flow" within Taiji creates the possibility of entering into the yellow chamber and into the enlightened state of Chin Hua.

It is necessary to use this backward flowing process to utilize those yin aspects of the energy system. To use ting jing and the relaxed state of song it is necessary to operate within the water path of the energy system. This places the adept in closer contact with po, which is necessary, in that the effort must be made to bring po and hun in closer connection with each other. The closer hun and po are to each other and the more in synchronization they are, then the higher the pitch in the vibration that is felt within the body. This vibration can attain the high pitch sounds of electrical transmission wires stretched under freezing temperatures. This high-pitched singing of high-tension wires is comparable to the sensations within the body when qi is elevated. The body literally sings with the infusion of this energy. The tinnitus that many people suffer from may be no more than this infusion of energy and the resultant inner sensations of the singing of this energy. It is the ego-mind aspect of hun that seeks preeminence and is aware of this close proximity of po, and seeks to regain its preeminence by medical means. The apparent cure for tinnitus would be removal or at the least diminishment of po if it were accomplished.

This vibration is the result of the close proximity of po and hun. It is called the "dragons hum and tiger's roar." This is what we seek. When they are working in close proximity and in unison, that is when we feel most alive. It is also when we can most directly access po and therefore utilize the energy system for martial purposes. The energy system of the body is much more complex than this, but for martial purposes, this limited understanding is all that is necessary at the moment.

4-5 Utilizing Kinesthetic Sensations.

Kinesthetic sensations and motor proprioceptor sensory stimuli can be used to develop this connection from the ground all the way through the body to the hand that is expressing power. Kinesthetic sensations involve the perception of the changes in the angle of the joints. This gives us a sense of movement, weight, and position. The proprioceptors receive stimuli within the tissues of the body as within the muscles and tendons.

The first and probably most important aspect is the kinesthetic sensations derived from the employment of the nine pearls. If you have done everything else right and have not connected the nine pearls, then the energy will be stopped at the first defective pearl. In order for the energy to move freely through the body the nine pearls must be all connected. The exercise standing like a tree or zhan zhuang, a qi gong exercise, is used to make you aware of some of the sensations of the nine pearls when they are connected. These specific pearls are; the wrist; the elbow; the shoulder and the ming men, (the gate of life) opposite the lower aspect of the sternum. The trick is to practice the rotation of the thumbs away from the body from this position and that of the compression of the ball, until those sensations can be duplicated without the postures. With the hands in front of the sternum (jade lady's hand), palms facing your chest, press the thumbs forward until pressure is felt at the joints and then with the palms rotated facing forward press the thumbs forward. If you are aware of the sensations and can pinpoint the proper locations, then you can learn to contract them at will, without contracting the muscles associated with them. This is necessary because with the advent of the wave of relaxation, it is necessary to maintain the connection of the nine pearls while allowing the controlled relaxation of the long muscles of the energy path. The contractions are with the muscle attachments to the tendons and the tendon and ligament attachments to the bone. It is not contraction of the large muscles of the body. It is the firming up of the connections or pearls, not a rigid immobilization of the structures.

The contraction of the long muscles on the storage phase of the fa jin cycle and the contraction of the nine pearls sequentially as the energy is drawn inward to the ground, allows the completion of these connections as the energy is stored. This sequential inward contraction of muscles and tendons gives one the sensation of movement through the body. If you understand the sequence of inward storage of energy and the sequential contractions, then you will understand the reversal, which is a sequential upward pressure along this compressed path until the ming men is passed and an outward exhalation releases the contractions of the long muscles, but not those of the nine pearls. It takes practice to relax one and not the other. It is also necessary to understand that the yongchuan is strummed with the nine pearls connected and the long muscles plus chan sichou in contraction. This makes it one piece through which the pulse can travel from the yongchuan through the first five pearls up to the ming men, where the breath is released and the long muscle contractions are released. This pulse is actively pushed through the six pearls and with the release, and the pulse is allowed to flow through the remaining contracted three pearls.

It is important to practice these sensations separate from the actual practice of fa jin so that the proper sequence is obtained. Without this proper sequence and nine pearls there is a very good chance that the energy will rebound to the first unconnected pearl and discharge the energy there. Considering the potential size of the force, it would be unwise to let this happen.

The contractions and sensations of chan sichou are the result of the twisting of muscle groups by the rotational movement of the body. This involves proprioceptor receptors of the muscle and tendons. It involves the long muscles of the legs (calf and thigh), the waist, and the forearm. The twisting due to the rotation of the waist in the storage phase of the fa jin cycle results in the storage of energy in the same manner as a twisted children's swing when released unwinds and releases this energy. This pulse, along with the strumming of the yongchuan, is delivered to the ming men point on the back, and from there it is released and song is prevalent as the pulse is pushed to the fingertips It is important to be very much aware of the existence of the nine pearls, and the contractions of the muscles as well as the strumming of the yongchuan. With this taut connection, the pulse released by the strumming of the yongchuan can be followed through the nine pearls and the contracted musculature released on its arrival at the ming men. These are sensations that must be followed and properly sequenced for the natural flow of the pulse of energy.

It is necessary to feel this pulse of energy as it moves through the body. It will not necessarily travel very fast through the body until it reaches the ming men and is released there. There are other forces, which accelerate the pulse, and these will be discussed individually.

4-6 Body Alignment and the Movement of Qi

In order for qi or the energy pulse of jin to move through the body, specific alignments must be met. To move through the shoulder and arm area of the body, it is necessary to use the configuration called beautiful lady's hand by the Chinese. It is called this because of the graceful natural curve of the arm and forearm. This natural curve allows the energy to move freely through this section of the body without the loss of energy. This graceful alignment of the structures allows the storage of borrowed energy from the opponent. The bio-kinetic pulse of jin requires the connection of joints and the specific alignments of the beautiful lady's hand to move without restriction through these areas. The flow of qi will be disrupted if the alignment is not accurate, and instead of flowing smoothly, it will be dispersed into the unaligned area, thus losing its martial value, and it results in the release of considerable energy in a local area.

The proper placement of the rear foot is critical. This is because there will be a loss of chan sichou if the angle is too wide, and a loss of song if the angle is too narrow. The torsion of chan sichou works best when there is a free articulation or the rotation of the joints on the plane of the force. Transfer of energy across all joints is affected if one joint is out of alignment.

The hip must be vertically in alignment with the rear foot so that it is centered over the heel of the foot at the beginning of fa jin. This alignment of the hip and rear foot is critical to the transfer of energy up to the waist. It is as if the bones were stacked one on top of each other like the plates in a jugglers act, over the heel of the rear foot. The energy must be able to move freely from the yongchuan to the ming men point for delivery to the fingertips. In order for this to happen, the hip must be thrust forward at this point in the transfer of energy, so that the spine can remain in an upright condition. Any leaning will result in tension of muscle groups to support the portion that is not aligned vertically. It is not possible to be song if muscle tension is created by unnecessary tension produced by leaning. It also results in discharge of force at an unusual angle and can result in a reduction of force, or return of energy to one of the nine pearls.

The forward thrust of the hips is done with the spine in a vertical position and it is carried forward, until the energy of fa jin is emitted while the spine remains vertical. There are many reasons for this. The main reason is that the head is oriented vertically and serves as a centering for the visual field so that opponents can be placed geometrically in the visual field with the same orientation for quicker analysis. It is po's ability to react to this geometric matrix that is critical to martial intentions.

The head and body must be in alignment so that there is a smooth transition of energy through the head region. In a karate punch, there is a noticeable snap of the head due to delivery of energy up the spine to the head region. The energy release from fa jin is so great that it is not advisable to release energy in this area. In karate, the release would be in the musculature of the head region, primarily in the stern-cleido-mastoideus muscles. The release of fa jin would occur in the muscle attachments and at the joints of the cervical spinal structure. It is necessary to push the energy through the ming men so that little of it actually is misdirected to the head region. Placement of the tongue on the palate serves to transfer a portion of any misdirected energy that does arrive at the head region up the back and also across the tongue bridge, and this divergence to the back and also the front of the head results in a final convergence at the top of the head which results in destructive interference and loss of energy that essentially neutralizes the energy wave in this area. The result is a considerably reduced wave front that is controlled by the splitting of the force into two channels and which is further contained by activating the cranial pump.

Blockage or release of energy in the lumbar area of the spine can result in the pumping action of the kidneys. This will lead to severe pain in the kidney area that greatly resembles the pain of kidney stones. It is for this reason that conscious effort must be made to push the energy through a perfectly aligned spinal column. This is an active push using the sacral pump and the qi belt

4-7 Centering and the Movement of Qi

There are several concepts relating to the center. One is maintaining the center, and the second is keeping the center. There is a third concept, which is remaining in the center. Maintaining the center is the effort involved in keeping the mind on the tantien such that all movement originates from this center. This has the effect of lowering your center of gravity and all movements have the characteristic of a spider in which all movement appears to be from one central point. This is a feeling that must be cultivated at all times.

Remaining in the center is picking the most advantageous spot and remaining there so that you are the center of all forces and all energy incoming and outgoing moves around you and through you, depending on the particular technique you are employing. This also must be cultivated at all times.

Keeping the center refers to the effort that must be used to orient your connecting extremity with the center line of your body in such a manner as to create an alignment between your center, your hand or other extremity and the center line of the opponent. This alignment should be on or parallel to a line drawn from the centerline of the front of your body to the centerline of the opponent's body. The directional arrow of the flow of qi will be along this line. This will have the effect of moving his centerline as if pressing directly on it, even though you are in reality pressing on his arm. You are manipulating his center and moving through his center by your attachment to his arm. The release of qi in fa jin has the same effect. The application of fa jin in the direction he is moving will be added to his movement. The release of fa jin at an appropriate angle can topple him in addition to the internal damage that can result.

The direction of the movement of qi determines the effect the qi has on the opponent. Even though the application is not on the center, the effect is the same as if it were directly applied to the centerline of the opponent as long as the force is moving in the direction of the center. The opponent will be pushed or force applied as if he was one piece and movement of one section moves him as if he was one integral piece. This is the reason rigidity of stance is not recommended.

If you are rigid in your stance and you are double weighted, then you are easily manipulated.

The proper alignment of the body in stepping is also critical. If you move in stepping as is normally done, then you will be free falling until contact is made with the ground and then an upward thrust against the floor is necessary to compensate for this acceleration. It is possible to manipulate the individual while he is in free fall or floating by the application of a minimum of force. This increases the downward acceleration and results in overcompensation, which results in the individual hopping. This has the effect of breaking his root with no apparent effort on your part. While the opponent is in mid air from the bounce that he received from the application of qi, it is then possible to an jin or fa jin the opponent with effective results.

4-8 Principles of Taiji Energy Movement

Muscular activity results in the accumulation of qi within the active muscles. This is called local qi, and it has some martial purposes. This type of energy is quickly dissipated and is replenished only by muscular activity. The internal movement of qi is not dependent on utilizing the muscles other than perhaps for storage purposes in the production of jing. Qi cannot be directly manipulated by the hun or wisdom mind aspect of this duality of mental existence. Qi is within the province of po. In order to move qi within the body, it is necessary to access po. All the training in Taiji is directed toward creating this accessibility to po in order to be able to use the energy. The slowness of the Taiji form, the visualizations, fighting sequences, interception and various other training methods are geared toward bringing hun and po in close proximity so that this accessibility is pre-eminent.

The first step in training this accessibility is to utilize the availability of local qi. We know that when muscles are contracted qi will flow into that area. It is possible then to create a flow of qi by contracting muscles sequentially so that the qi will follow a specific sequence of a wave front produced by the contractions of the muscles. This is much like creating a furrow from a mud puddle and the water flows to fill in the void left behind by the stick. The difficulty in moving qi lies in the fact there is no sensory feedback from the movement of qi. The effects of qi can be seen but the more the effect is from qi and not jing, then, the less effort is felt in producing the effect. There is no rebound of energy on the release when striking as there is in fa jin. It is an immediate soft release of energy in which you are not even aware of the energy contained within the release.

The classics state that the yi leads the qi (yi yi yin qi). This indicates the fact that the hun or wisdom mind, much as the stick drawn through the sand leads the water on a winding course, leads by means of visualization techniques and various sensory manipulations the qi on a course through the body for martial purposes. A good example of this process is the classic statement that "you must adhere the qi to the back." Knowing that local qi resides in the active muscles, allows you to move qi through the back by sequentially contracting the spinal attachments of the ligaments of the spinalis dorsi, longissimus dorsi and the sacro spinalis muscles at the back area. The sensory feedback from the muscle groups facilitates this movement. You can be aware of the muscle contractions and be certain that the local qi is moving with this sequential muscular contraction. As you accumulate qi within the body, by various methods, this too will move with the local qi when you are actively moving the local qi.

Actively moving the local qi assists in the alignment of structures, and creation of the nine pearls. This facilitates the movement of qi. It is through the sensory feedback derived from active muscular groups that we can increase the flow of qi. We do not directly sense the flow of qi, but like the metal filings in a magnetic field, we can see the results and the peripheral effects.

4-9 Threading the Qi

The qi moves through the body along a prescribed path for martial purposes. It is possible to fill the body with qi for health purposes, but in the martial arena, it is necessary to move it from the rooted rear foot through the various nine pearls, through the sacral pump to the qi belt, adhere it to the spine and then deliver it to the fingertips. This connection is visualized as a silk thread that moves through the body from the strummed rear foot to the fingertips. All of these connections (nine pearls) must be made prior to the strumming of the rear foot during the storage phase.

To make all the connections it is necessary to reverse the visualization during the storage phase and visualize the silk thread moving from the fingertips through the wrist, elbow, shoulder to the ming men point down the back, reversing the muscular contractions with a downward flow at the back, relaxing the sacral pump and then through the remainder of the nine pearls, until you have reached the yongchuan point on the ball of the rear foot. It is important that you do not press down on the yongchuan point. The proper way to strum the rear foot is to press it in such a manner that you are lifting the body, rather than pressing your weight into the floor. The difference is that to reach an object on an upper shelf, the upward thrust lifts you, whereas if you had your foot on someone and were trying to keep them down, you would then be pressing down on the floor, using different muscular force with greater intensity. This is a soft and gentle lifting of the body, an almost imperceptible lift.

All of the connections that were made by the storage phase with reverse visualization of the movement of the silk thread of qi must be held and remain intact as you reverse the process so that this silk thread is actively felt as you move the pulse formed by the strumming of the rear foot up through the nine pearls.

The threading of qi is critically important during the storage phase. This is a visualization that will set up the continuity of the various segments of the body. This occurs prior to release of the energy pulse.

4-10 Release of the Qi in Martial Applications

The storage phase of the threading of the qi is essential because this is what sets up the continuity of the bodily structures so that the pulse can move through those places of constriction and those places of discontinuity, either of which will prevent the flow of qi through these areas. Considering the amount of energy moving through the body, it is essential that a free flow of energy be possible at all times. This requires a mental effort that is not a usual accompaniment to martial purposes. The reverse threading of the qi visualizations for this continuity must become a part of the training sequence so that they occur each time fa jin training is attempted.

If the release of energy at the fingertips is not complete, the energy will rebound and express itself at the first restriction or discontinuous pearl (joint). The release must occur without loss of continuity; without constriction caused by muscular effort; song must be evident; the breathing must lead the pulse and the air expelled with the pulse at the ming men point.

The pulse generated by the downward pressure at the yongchuan point is actively pushed through the body. This push follows the breath and it is an active manipulation of the pulse through the body. Each individual segment of the pulse must have its accompanying continuity and kinesthetic feedback so that you have song (a relaxed sentience) and the proper connections at the same time. This requires being relaxed in the musculature, but connected at the pearls by contraction of the muscle attachments at the joints. This pulse must be manipulated by the mind with a sequencing of a contraction that yields the feeling of a push following the breath and leading the kinesthetic sensation of qi moving through the body. It is not the qi that is being felt, but rather the pressure at the yongchuan the release of chan sichou at the leg muscles the twisting; the forward thrust of the hips; the compression at the qi belt; the sacral pump; adhering to the spine and finally the release of breath at the ming men with the push to the fingertips.

The release at the fingertips is accomplished by the forceful stopping of the forward movement of the hand. This results in the accumulation of this force in the fingertips. If the hand is a knife hand with a straight forward projection, then the energy accumulated results in the forward movement of the finger joints as if someone were pulling the last joint forward in the direction of the release. If the hand is in the peng position with the hand perpendicular to the forward motion, then pulse is released with a hinge movement of the joints in the fingers and the hand. This is where the concept of the beautiful lady's hand comes into play. This is the graceful arc from the shoulder to the fingertips that must be maintained in the release of energy in fa jin and an jin. If this is not maintained, then the hand, fingers and wrist act separately as if hinged. Not only is there a loss of power, but the energy will rebound and whip the joints causing injury over time. The fingertips, wrist, elbow and shoulder are particularly vulnerable because the energies reach a maximum as the qi approaches these areas. If you experience discomfort or soreness in these areas, examine yourself for the nine pearls, song, beautiful lady's hand and a push of the energy rather than a whipping of the energy.

The release must allow the free rebound of energy. Any rigidity in structure will create a stoppage of energy release of whole body power. The hand and foot must always arrive together. This can be practiced at the candle. You are admonished by the classics to place your foot, heel first, in most instances. This is an effort to coordinate hand and foot. It allows you to position your leg and foot so that weight can then be moved over the forward leg and the coordination can then occur.

4-11 The Use of Qi in Health Applications

The movement of the qi through the body by means of fa jin can be used also for manipulating the energy system of the body. There are advanced methods of moving the qi through the body. These will be discussed later, but for now the basic difference at this level is that the release in fa jin is an abrupt stoppage of the rapidly moving hand so that the energy is released in an explosive pulse. The release for health applications is a soft stop such that the qi rolls off the fingertips in a continuous flow of energy over a much longer period of time. The effect is very noticeable at the candle in lazhu fangfa. The release in fa jin results in an explosive extinguishing of the candle, however, with the soft release the candle is put out by a steady flow of energy with as much or more explosive power, but no accompanying rebound of the extremity. This is a noticeable difference that surprises you when it happens. It is an effortless endeavor that is a striking contrast to the rebound of the hand in fa jin. It is puzzling when it first happens, because there is a lack of feedback, which would tell you the release is complete. It is as if this energy left the hand before the whole process was completed. This is, however, the energy we seek to demonstrate within the techniques of Taiji. It is the ultimate goal of the martial aspects of Taiji. It is of concern at this time to learn to produce fa jin, since this is more easily obtained for martial purposes. In our attempts to produce fa jin, we will be concurrently developing some movement of qi within the body. This will also assist in the development of the movement of qi for health purposes.

Section Two:
Energy Storage

5

Basic Energy Development

5-1 Qi Gong and Its Relationship

Around ten thousand years ago, in the beginnings of civilization, a keenly obser-vant shaman understood that the Great Dance, called Da Wu in Chinese, granted the participants important health benefits, especially for those that engaged in the Great Dance. It was a communal tribal dance, at first only cere-monial in nature and was considered the province of the tribal shaman. The strength, energy and vitality of the ceremonial dancers increased from their par-ticipation in the da wu. The Yellow Emperor's Classic of Internal Medicine expressed this ancient practice and led to the creation of qi gong as it. This docu-mentation of the art of qi gong occurred in the first and second centuries BC.

During this era, it was discovered that these exercises were of tremendous use in applying martial forces. The external styles that existed at the time quickly adapted them into their practices. The Taoist in the meantime discovered inter-nal techniques for the movement of qi through the body. Through the centuries, qi gong became an integral part of the martial applications of this internal energy and movement of this intrinsic force within the body. The similarity between the forms of Taiji and the internal and the external qi gong set of postures is not coincidental. The static and dynamic postures and forms of Taiji are designed in a manner that specifically allows the movement of qi through the body with a minimum of force so that it is possible to go from a state of relaxed sentience or song to one of maximum force or fa jin, and then back to song. The effectiveness of moving in a state of song results from the methods of stature and posture inherent in the qi gong training. Qi gong is a form of standing meditation and Taiji is a method of moving meditation. It is a means of transferring qi through various postures with stepping, without losing the flow of qi to the extremities. This relationship between qi gong and the internal martial arts has been constant down through the ages.

5-2 Fang Song Gong

Relaxation as defined by the term song is not the limp, total relaxation one achieves with massage, but is instead a relaxed sentience that results from the use of minimal muscular effort in maintaining posture or movement that eliminates unnecessary muscular tension. The result is an unimpeded movement that can sustain itself over longer periods of time, because the energy expended is minimal.

The term fang song gong transliterates as "method of relaxed effort," which is a very good definition of what is required to be song. Relaxed sentience is using no more effort than necessary to maintain posture and alertness as to what is occurring outside you. Most battles are lost in that period of time before a battle in which the waiting is very destructive to mind and body. Elevated tension can deplete the energy of the warrior before the battle begins. It is hun the ego-mind that takes the warrior into emotionally charged areas that result in increased tension. It is po that removes one from the ten thousand things and delivers you into this serene state of the eternal now. It is the past that is emotionally charged and it is the future that is filled with apprehension. Po does not operate within the domain of language and conceptual thinking, therefore, it does not have a concept of past or future, and therefore it does not operate within these domains.

It is the practice of qi gong that teaches the novice how to maintain posture and move energy through the body without the expenditure of excessive amounts of energy. It is by way of training to control and balance the forces within the body that this serene sentience po is attained at the proper moment in a conflict. Much of the training within Taiji is the mental development of the means of accessing po.

5-3 Qi Gong Exercises

There are specific ways of doing various qi gong exercises that are of primary importance to lazhu fangfa. For instance, the Zhang Zhuang exercise "standing like a post" does many different things for the internal artist, if it is done in a specific way. (see figure 4)

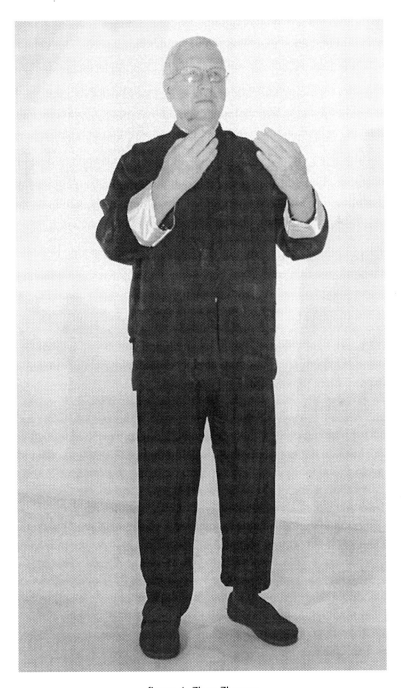

figure 4. Zhan Zhuang

This exercise is begun in the ma pu stance and then the arms are moved into a position as if holding a large ball against your chest. To train for fa jin, there are various things that must be added to the stance internally to gain from this exercise.

The exercise is begun with an inward breath as if drawing through a straw. This should be felt as a contraction in the tantien area. This is "reverse Taoist breathing." Visualization is an important part of this exercise, and must accompany it in order to be successful. The first visualization is to follow the breath (inhale) for ming jing and an jing from the tips of your fingers on the right hand through the nine pearls down to the ming men through the spine and down to the heel and to the yongchuan of the left foot. Return the breath (exhale) for ming jing (visible force) and an jing (invisible force) and (inhale) for hua jing (perfect force) from the yongchuan of the left foot to the fingertips of the right hand. Repeat this exercise on the left, beginning with the left hand.

The second exercise, still from the Than Zhuang exercise "standing like a post," move your hands with your thumbs pointing toward the ceiling, to a position rotated forward so that your thumbs are at a forty five-degree angle pointing away from your body. This should been done on inhale as if breathing through a straw and at the same time the hands are rotated so the thumb is pointing down. The thumbs are then pressed forward so that the thumbs are at a forward angle of approximately forty five-degrees.

While holding this last posture, move your hands slightly apart and at the same time inward toward the body. This should be accompanied by an inhale, and as before, there should be a sensation of tension at the shoulder and the scapular attachment at the spinal column. Accompanying this exercise, should be the visualization that the ball is expanding in size creating this movement and you are resisting. It is important to visualize this sensation as something that is happening to you, and that the effort to accomplish this task be minimal.

The object is to create tension in a segment of the nine pearls such that only enough tension is felt so that they can be identified. It is proper to minimize the tension in the rest of the body so that you are song. A rigid connection of the nine pearls is not necessary. Excessive tension can only hinder movement. The movement of the body from yin to yang and back in an instant cannot be accomplished if you are not song.

This particular qi gong stance is effective for rooting practice which is very relevant for Taiji practice.

5-4 Qi Gong and Breath Development

Within the gentle sound of the inhale, there exists the visualization that ties all this together. It is by means of this soft drift of the breath that we can coordinate all things martial. As previously mentioned, the water follows the line drawn in the sand as described and this is a perfect metaphor for the movement of qi through the meridians of the body as a deliberate tensioning and relaxation threads through the body, causing the qi to flow in its path.

The "standing like a post" posture of qi gong is for external arts merely a strengthening exercise. It has a more significant part to play for the internal arts. In addition to the strengthening aspects of qi gong, the breathing is done in a manner that facilitates the flow of qi. The seemingly unrewarding long periods of the qi gong posture standing like a post allows one to practice threading the qi through the body. This creates the conceptual idea of a groove through which qi can flow. The more times you do this exercise, the less effort will be required. It will occur without the practitioner having to force the qi through the body. It becomes a natural movement (ziran) that occurs when it is required.

By following this thin silk thread of the breath, our mind is on the activity, and our ego-mind is bored and seeks escape. It is by virtue of our resolve to stay within the qi gong parameters that we defeat the incessant demands of the ego-mind. Po becomes pre-eminent and we have accomplished a major transitional point forward in our martial development. The thread that ties these together is the form; lazhu fangfa; the techniques, and the reality of the street is the breath and its visualization as a thread of silk. These simple exercises may seem trivial, but they can have a large impact on your performance.

5-5 The Qi Belt and Energy Movement

The movement of the waist using the large muscles of the body is a problem for most Taiji students. It is a troublesome location for the flow of qi through the body since it consists mostly of soft tissue and muscle. All loosely connected parts of the body must be integrated so that the connection for the upward thrust of qi from the yongchuan through the turning of the waist and the forward thrust of the hips and with reverse Taoist breathing can be combined to move smoothly through this area without any loss. Rebound in this area is problematic. The kidneys will pump up and down like pistons, causing a very painful condition that feels like kidney stones. Particular effort must be made to move the qi through this area without dissipation of energy in the soft tissues.

The qi belt itself does not comprise the muscles in the belt area, but instead consists of the compression of this area by reverse Taoist breathing; compression by the movement of the diaphragm down in front and up in back; contraction and tensing of the fascia, and the actuation of the sacral pump. The energy is actively pushed through this area by this compression that yields pneumatic and hydraulic pressures in this area. Care must be taken not to exert excessive force in delivering energy through this area. It only requires a boost through this area, not an increase of energy. There are too many soft tissues in this area that can be damaged by excessive use of force.

5-6 The Sacral Pump and Energy Movement

The sacrum is a fused piece of bone, triangular in shape that is located at the base of the spine. There is a restriction of movement forward and backward in this segment of the spine. Ligament and muscle attachments here permit minimal movement. With practice, contractions in this area in conjunction with the qi belt will assist in the movement of qi through this area of difficult qi movement. It is much like the squeezing of a tube of toothpaste. A constant pressure applied at the proper moment in this area causes the qi to move effortlessly through this area.

To practice this technique and acquire the proper sensations, lie down with your back to the floor. With subtle movement of the sacral area, it is possible to lift the pelvic girdle a small distance off the floor. The movement and its sensations will come with practice.

5-7 The Cranial Pump and Energy Movement

The cranial pump along with the tongue pressed against the teeth to form a connection allows qi to pass through the forward aspect of the head in addition to the surge up the back of the head. These two forces are neutralized by destructive interference when they meet. This results in reducing the tension required by the shoulder muscles to steady the head when the force rebounds as in the external styles. An important characteristic of the hard styles is this forceful snap of the head with the forward thrust of the striking hand.

While rhythmically clenching the teeth, feel in the temporal region with your fingers for the contraction of these muscle groups. This should identify the cranial pump. Tension in the stern-cleido-mastoideus muscles inhibits the flow of qi from the ming men point to the shoulder. It is important also to steady the head so that awareness of the surrounding environment is not impeded. Taiji as an internal art demands that every effort be made to ensure that awareness of your surroundings and the ability to move is not blocked by increased tension or misalignment of the body.

The contraction of these muscles serves to reduce the flow of energy through this region and as a result, the rebound of energy creating tension in the sternocleido-mastoideus muscles is reduced. Relax the shoulders is an important part of the Taiji ability to be song, because the total body must be relaxed, not just certain portions.

5-8 Rotating the Qi Ball in the Tantien

Conceptually there exists two separate cycles to the visualized rotation of the qi ball. One cycle occurs on the inhale or storage phase of the cycle and the other occurs on the exhale or emission stage of the cycle. The qi ball is located in the abdominal area, and it is the rotation of this conceptual ball that results in the movement of qi through this soft tissue area on the storage and emission phases of fa jin.

On inhale, the ball is visualized rotating downward on the front side so that there is a feeling of compression in the lower abdominal area. This results in the storage of energy in the muscles and fascia of the abdominal area, and compresses the energy in the lower segment of the body. This sequence is done for ming jing (visible force) and an jing (hidden force) and the inhale and exhale are reversed in hua jing (perfect force).

When the cycle of breathing reverses from storage to emission, the compression and movement of energy is thrust upward along the inner side of the spinal column to the ming men, this in combination with the qi belt and sacral pump will move the qi through this area, and it will add additional energy to the pulse of qi moving through the body. This pressure on the movement of qi must be a constant throughout the body so that the continuity is not broken. One technique for moving the qi through the body must not end before control has been taken over by the next method.

The qi gong exercise rolling the golden ball in conjunction with reverse Taoist breathing is an excellent exercise to gain control over this process of turning the Taiji ball. It is essential that the breath is coordinated with the direction of the spin of the ball. The tantien must be visualized as a golden ball and in front of the tantien; the hands are holding a duplicate visualized golden ball. The hands will make circular motions in front of the tantien as if you were holding a ball and rotating it outward, downward, inward and then upward. The breathing coordination is as follows: inhale as the ball is moved outward; the tantien is contracted downward as the ball moves downward; the ball is moved inward and exhale begins and the breath pushes upward with relaxation at the end. The downward segment of the rotation cycle is coordinated with the downward movement of the diaphragm in the tantien area. Practice in this can greatly enhance your fa jin capabilities.

5-9 The Energy Centers of the Body

The energy centers of the body, particularly the three tantien, are of importance to lazhu fangfa and the internal martial arts because of their implementation in the production of qi, and their usage in inculcating the concept of song in a conflict, of the need for access to po in a conflict situation. (see figure 5) The first of these centers is called the Zhang tantien or upper tantien.

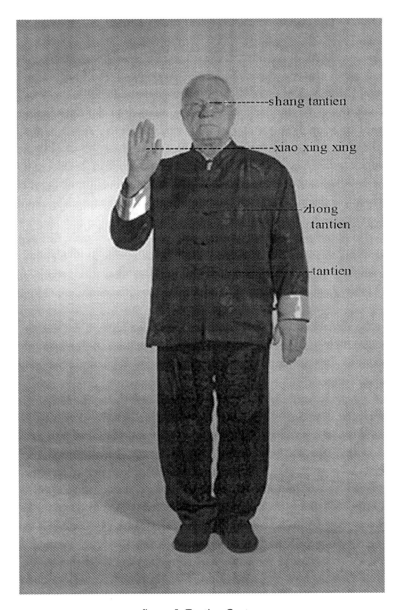

figure 5. Tantien Centers

It is located at the third eye or pineal gland mid point in the brain. It is called the yellow door, golden chamber or yellow room in various Chinese arts. The lower tantien is called xiao tantien. It is also called the sea of qi or xiaohai in Chinese medicine. The middle tantien is called zhong tantien, and it is located in the solar plexus.

The lower tantien, or sea of qi, is considered for martial and health purposes as the source of qi that can be manipulated throughout the body. The Chinese believe that the abdomen must be made to move continually in and out in order to replenish the qi in the body in the same manner as the fetus pumps blood throughout its body. It is not that qi is created within this area but that circulation of the qi in the twelve meridians results in concentration of qi in some area and results less in other areas. By moving the abdomen in breathing as a baby does, the circulation will be maintained, and the distribution of qi will be uniform. There are twelve qi channels or meridians through which qi moves from the various organs to the extremities. There are eight reservoirs of qi in addition to the twelve meridians and they serve as storage of qi. They must be full, and the free flow from them to the meridians must be maintained. These eight vessels regulate the flow of qi within the meridians, and therefore it is essential that they be full. The two major vessels that have martial concern are the conception vessel and the governing vessel. The conception vessel is yin and is on the front of the body on the centerline, and runs from the top of the head to the hui yin located at the perineum (the base of the torso) where it then joins the governing vessel. It then moves to the top of the head, at this point it joins the conception vessel completing the loop.

The fire path is from the tantien up the back and down the front. The water path is a reverse direction of the flow. The practice of Taiji and qi gong can result in the body becoming too yang, if there is an over abundance of yang techniques. When it is said that the body is too yang, it means that the body is operating within the active principle, it is energetic, full of qi and intent on doing something. It is the state of hun, the ten thousand things, the active yang principle the wisdom mind (yi) that is predominant. It is necessary to cool down the body if it becomes too yang for an excessively long period of time. If the body is in continuous yang condition, the body is then placed in an enduringly stressful situation that can lead to damage to the body. Reducing the yang condition of the body is achieved by entering into the state of po. The yin principle predominates within po, and it is the inactive, dark yielding condition that is pre-eminent.

If you are song, then no harm will come to the body. The trick is to be song so that you are always prepared, yet you have immediate access to the lower tantien for martial purposes. Practice in the form and qi gong will teach you how to remain in a state of existence, which borders on hun and po so that access is immediate from one to the other. This is the balanced state required for combat.

The ten thousand things are not evident and we are not lost within the geometric matrix of po. The wisdom mind of hun leads the activity, but it leads with a narrow focus. It is almost as if one were oscillating between the two, with hun or the wisdom mind aspect of it, leading po in the martial arena. It is access to po that we seek. It is not the focus of this practice to remain within po, but it is the necessity of having immediate access to it. It is po, which has access to the energy systems within the body. Hun is able to use them only through this balance and proximity with po.

The lower tantien is of primary use in martial energy. It is called the sea of qi or qihai in Chinese. The middle tantien is the solar plexus and heart area. Breathing exercises in the tumo tradition of Tibet can enhance song. It is possible to be totally relaxed within the musculature of the body and still not be song. To be song you must also relax the vascular system of the body so that there is a free flow of fluids to the organs, the brain and the musculature of the body. A test of whether you are song is the temperature of your hands. If they are cold, or even cool, then you are not song, even if you are totally relaxed. Proper breath control can lead you into this state of song. This is not a yang state, in which you have placed qi in your hands as in fa jin, but is instead a yin state in which you have relaxed the musculature of the vaso-constrictors so that the free flow of blood is evident.

To accomplish the breathing into your hands technique, draw in a breath with the accompanying visualization of attempting to blow on the glowing embers of tinder as if you were starting a fire in the woods. Too strong a breath and you will blow out the glowing tinder. There must be enough breath to fan the tinder but not enough to cause it to extinguish. Visualize the tinder diminishing as you draw in a breath and increasing in a red glow as you breathe out. This is breath control, and as you fan the fire on exhale, you visualize this fire breath extending down to your hands so that they feel the warmth of the ever increasing fanning of the embers. These embers should be visualized as existing in the heart area of the upper tantien

This is a simple exercise, but its effects are considerable. It is through this relaxation of the vaso-constrictors that one can be proficient in the reduction of high blood pressure and much of the anxiety and tension that accompanies life in the western culture. With relaxed tension and anxiety, this state of balance between hun and po is more evident.

For martial purposes in fa jin, you will breathe from and move from the lower tantien. For purposes of song and the preparatory exercise, you will breath with the middle tantien.

There are various sensory aspects that serve as a precursor to a conflict. The first stage is the awareness of the eminent onset of the conflict. This is a time when you must be song and breathe warmth into your hands. To fa jin requires "reverse Taoist breathing" and the breath comes from the lower tantein. This must be trained so that it is naturally occurring and becomes a part of the technique. If you are intent on applying a technique, it will not work. You must follow the energy and allow the proper technique to happen.

The actual triggering event within the conflict should immediately launch you into the state of po so that you can marshal the energy forces that po has under its command. In addition to qi, there is the sensory ability of ting jing, while in contact with the opponent. When you are not physically engaged or in the initial confrontation before you are in contact, sensory abilities are available from the upper tantien. This is considered the seat of the soul. It is located within the pineal gland, which is located approximately mid brain. These abilities are extra-sensory and obtained only with great difficulty, but they are available for those who train with dedication. These abilities are not separate and distinct from normal abilities but stretch along a continuum in which the more deeply you are involved in the state of po, the more remarkable are the powers you can obtain. At the ultimate, these powers are not available when you are in within the yi mind but occur in the trance-like state of po.

5-10 Small Universe Circulation

The movement of qi within the body along prescribed paths has martial applications. It is possible to concentrate qi in the tantien for use in fa jin when the necessity arises. This ensures that a reservoir of qi is available on demand. Otherwise, local qi will be depleted almost immediately. This storage in the tantien is very much like squeezing a long thin balloon. The air is removed from the middle and concentrates in the ends and the ends expand to a larger size. It is possible to do this because the qi has difficulty moving through the hui yin in the perineum and must be intentionally and actively forced through this area. This resistance to the flow of qi allows the practitioner to accumulate qi in the tantien area for later martial usage.

The small universe circulation leaves the tantien, goes through the pelvic area, up the spine through the neck and head area, and returns to the tantien. Areas of restriction and difficult passage for qi are; the hui yin point on the perineum; the ming men which is on the spine in back across from the sternum; the jade pillow yuzhen which is at the back of the head; the crown of the head baihui point and finally the brow point called the shang tantien or upper tantien.

To follow the movement of qi through the body, it is necessary to visualize the qi with some activity that has a feedback component. There is no sensory feedback to the movement of qi within the body. It is known, however, that the qi collects within the muscles and other tissue when activity occurs in that area. For instance, when a muscle group is flexed there will be an accumulation in the muscles that are active. It is possible to feel the flexing of the muscles and the heat generated in that area. If muscles are flexed in sequence, it is then possible to follow the flow of this energy of contraction and at the same time follow the movement of the qi as it accompanies this muscular flow of energy. It is through this means that we can follow the flow of qi and manipulate it to our purposes.

Small universe circulation along the fire path is a visualization technique in which the qi is made to follow the manipulations of the ego-mind aspect of hun by manipulating the musculature and by using breathing techniques. Compressing the diaphragm squeezes the qi through the hui yin point where it is moved up the spine by compression of the qi belt and the sacral pump. The muscle attachments of the ribs at the spine are contracted in sequence to move the qi further up to the ming men point. Instead of distributing to the fingertips, the qi is moved up to the "jade pillow" or the yuzhen point at the back of the head. This is the point on the back of the head, which is in contact with the floor if you were to rest there. It then is moved to the "crown point" or bai hui at the top of the head, then to the upper tantien, that point between the eyebrows, and then finally returned to the lower tantien. The utilization of muscle contractions is a means of identifying the movement of qi to enhance the sensations of qi moving through this circulation. These muscle contractions can be reduced when the visualization technique is in place. There will be minute muscular contractions as you advance that will allow you to follow the movement of qi. These subtle muscular movements can be trained with constant usage, and they gain in ability to move qi with usage. By placing our attention at various locations in the body, we are able to move qi into that area, and by moving the attention along a specific path, we also can move the qi along this path at the same speed as the attention is moving. This seemingly minor capacity to move qi by the subtle manipulation of the attention and muscular effort has major implications for martial arts and spiritual advancement.

5-11 Large Universe Circulation

The obvious distinction between the large and small universe circulations is the focal point of the energy distribution. Small circulation is limited to the conception and governing vessel. Within the large universe circulation, the energy is moved to every part of the body. Chinese literature states that the qi should be pushed to the ends of all the hairs. The martial implication of this is that you are filling the body with qi instead of returning and storing it in the tantien.

5-12 Ren Mai

The ren mai is also called the conception vessel. Its relevance for martial purposes is that it is an area that readily lends itself to perception of the movement of qi or the accompaniments of qi that assist in training for the movement of qi. It is also called the red line. The ease with which qi can be moved through this area makes it an important area of practice. To practice this, as you breathe in, visualize a red line moving upward from the tantien to the middle tantien.

5-13 The Seat of Fire and Water

Kan is the water element and it has the capacity to cool the body down, while li is the fire element and will result in higher body temperature. Kan and li are the means by which this occurs, while yin and yang is the end results of these efforts. The water element is used to cool down the fire element, but this cooling must not be so much that the fire mind is eliminated. The fire mind is active in life sustaining conditions, as all life would be extinguished without it. The fire qi creates the xin mind, and the yang mind or emotional mind. By cooling down the yang or xin mind, the yin or wisdom mind prevails within hun. Meditation and the techniques of Taiji increase the cooling effects of the yang mind and result in the preeminence of the wisdom mind as opposed to the xin or emotional mind.

This is of importance because it is the wisdom mind that is trained to lead the qi. The significance of this lies in the fact that it is po that moves the qi and it is by virtue of the developed proximity between the wisdom mind and po that this can occur. The nature of this relationship will be discussed later.

5-14 Cultivating the Qi

The qi utilized for martial purposes can be cultivated by various means. The most common uses by martial artists are still and moving meditation. The still meditation can be either standing or sitting. Standing meditation of the qi gong type is common within the Taiji community. Taiji itself is considered a moving meditation.

Everything you do is an opportunity to increase qi and develop this relationship between the yi mind and po. Every breath we take and every activity we engage in serves as an opportunity to exert force and move the qi at the same time. This can be done by reducing the effort necessary to move within the world by greatly reducing muscular effort and deliberately increasing the force of qi.

6

Storage of Energy within the Body

6-1 The First Bow of Posture

The bow and arrow was of critical importance in the martial arts and warfare. It is only natural that terms and training would carry over from one to the other. Terms such as stringing the bow, the bow, the arrow of direction and releasing qi like the release of an arrow are common in the Chinese striking arts. This imagery should assist in delivering the real art.

The first bow of posture is identified by the Chinese term mei ren shou or beautiful lady's hand. This is also called yu nu shou or jade lady's hand. This is a common position of the arms and hands within the Taiji stance called peng (see figure 6).

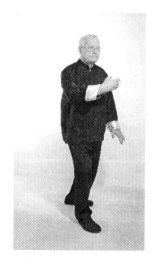

figure 6 Peng Posture

82

It is called this because of the graceful and delicate appearance of the rounded features of the hand, arm and forearm. These gradual curves serve as a means of storing energy, which can be released from various postures, peng being the most common. The energy resulting from compression, created by actively producing an inward force, by working opposing groups of muscles with a visualized inward intention, as if you were holding a ball on your chest and compressing it inward, creates an outward force when the inward force is released and the unopposed outward force is allowed to expend itself.

If you were to compress this imaginary ball inward using opposing muscles and then released only the inward force, there would then be an outward rebound which can be combined in a additive way with all fa jin derived forces.

The first bow is a recurved bow. Its form is identified by the hands at the side raised to a forward upright position level with the shoulders and the hand, palm facing inward, centered between the middle and lower tantien. A slight curvature at the elbow and the wrist gives this bow the appearance of a recurved bow. The tension developed by the additional curves of the bow, serve to add increased tension when the bow is strung. By using opposing muscles, it is possible to gain the same effect when each individual hand is moved into the nu yu shou position

6-2 The Second Bow of Posture

The second bow of posture consists of an arc that follows the rear foot up the rear leg to the hips, along the spine to the top of the head. This bow is strung using the archery metaphor by the turning of the waist. As with the first bow, the second bow is a device for the storage of energy by means of the compression of the muscles within the waist, leg and foot in the form of chan sichou, which is defined as silk reeling. It is derived from the Chinese art of removing the single continuous thread of silk from the silk worm cocoon. These two forces are combined with energy of the first bow in the first step of production of fa jin.

6-3 The Third Bow of Posture

The third bow is formed by the arch created by the rear leg connected through the hui yin point down the forward leg and culminating in the forward foot. This bow is activated by the forward thrusting of the hips and the force of gravity resulting from sinking the qi as the center of effort is moved over the forward foot.

6-4 Old Ox Power

This component of the energy cycle is named after the observation of animals, which is very common in the martial applications of force. In plowing fields with oxen, it was observed that when plowing ox encountered a root or heavy obstacle would plant its opposing feet, i.e. rear foot and opposing front foot. With the rope from the harness draped over its shoulder and across its waist, it would rotate its waist as it pressed forward. It was this movement by the waist that gave the tremendous force and power through this connection from rear foot to front foot. An ancient practice of old ox power utilized for thousands of years consists of standing on a rope with it stretched across your waist and over your shoulder to your upward outstretched hand, in the manner of the ox as it struggled with the load. With the rotation of your waist, your hand is moved by the connection made by the rope. The purpose of this practice is to internalize this connection without the use of the rope after a period of practice. Time and practice of this connection will, combined with the nine pearls, lead to old ox power, which is a unique form of whole body power or zhen jing. The difference between old ox power and peng is the direction of rotation of the waist with reference to the forward foot. With in peng with the right foot forward the rotation is clockwise. It is reversed for old ox power.

6-5 Chan Sichou

This is the energy developed from the rotation of the waist, which causes the energy to be stored within the stretched or compressed muscles of the leg and waist. It is likened to the removal of a single slender thread from the cocoon of the silk worm. Similarly, it takes a deliberate, delicate and continuous effort to remove that single strand of silk from the cocoon. The same uninterrupted and delicate threading of the qi through the body must occur if you are to deliver the qi from the yongchuan to the fingertips. This must be a delicate effort and a conscious effort to exert only enough force needed to remove the thread and yet, not too much effort or the thread will be broken. It is important to lead the thread without exerting enough force to break it, because this will result in substantial diminution of the power of chan sichou. That single thread of silk in the ancient process would be wound on a spindle as it is removed from the cocoon. The waist can be compared to the spindle, and as it is rotated, the thread is extracted from the cocoon, which is allowed to spin freely. The thread in this instance is the stored energy resulting from the initial turning of the waist, which results in the torsion in the muscle groups of the leg and waist. This is similar to a twisted rope, which is allowed to unwind. This, however, is a controlled unwinding. The energy is deliberately moved up pathways, through the nine pearls with conscious effort until it is expressed in the hand. It is very similar to squeezing a tube of toothpaste and moving the paste through the tube until it spurts out the end. With practice, it feels as if the qi is squeezed through the body and spurts out the hand. It is a sequencing of effort that moves the qi through the body. Chan sichou occurs in two parts. There is an initial storage phase and then the release phase. It is as if you compressed a spring from both ends and then slowly released the pressure on one end until the spring reached the target area and then was completely released. When the energy is stored and on release, it can be slowly moved from the yongchuan through the nine pearls as the muscular contractions deliver this pulse of energy derived from strumming the yongchuan.

6-6 Fa jin

Fajin is the energy delivered into the opponent. An explosive force is internally created and then delivered through the connected nine pearls until conveyed in martial form through the hands or extremities of the body. It is an intricately formed and released explosion of energy, and it has many facets that must be carefully coordinated, integrated and delivered without any discontinuity, or there will be considerable power loss. The beginning of this process is the storage phase; it initiates fa jin. The storage phase of fa jin is an elaborate convergence of forces. If you visualize the energy streaming in from the fingertips through the nine pearls to the yongchuan, you will quickly acquire the necessary connections. This is beneficial because it trains you to attend to the connections of the nine pearls, which are firmly connected during the storage phase that they are ready for energy emission prior to the second or the release phase of the delivery. It is not possible to make the nine pearls firm on the emission phase of fa jin and maintain the proper and important condition of being song.

Visualization is an important part of any technique in Taiji because it is a means of access to po. The fact that your attention is on various parts of your body to accomplish an elaborate sequence of events, initiates those specific things you have trained. The nine pearls, beautiful lady's hand, and postures are good examples of this. The storage phase is the preparatory sequence for emission of the energy pulse of fa jin. The storage phase allows the free flow of the energy pulse from the yongchuan to the fingertips without discontinuity.

The storage phase follows the inward movement of the breath, which combines with the inward contraction of the abdomen. This is reverse Taoist breathing. The breath then is drawn inward as a cool thin shaft of air, as if drawing through a straw. This is the yin phase and as such should be cool. The imagery of coolness will assist in accessing po and calming the mind in the face of the opponent. Much of the training in the walking meditation of Taiji is removing the ego from the combat scene and replacing it with po. This yin phase is the precursor for the release of qi. The release is also not a yang phase, although it may have yang elements, it is a yin activity. Po must be retained throughout the storage and emission phases of fa jin. The method of rolling the qi ball can be used here to facilitate the inward and outward expression of qi.

As the breath is drawn in, the waist is turned in the direction of the rear foot, causing the muscles of the leg and ankle to twist and compress, forming the energy of chan sichou. This rotation should make the position of the yongchuan point readily perceptible. It is by pressing down on the yongchuan that the process of fa jin emission begins.

This strumming of the yongchuan is not a downward press such as that which you would use to press someone to the floor, but it is instead a downward press that lifts the body. It is as if you were attempting to get something off the top shelf and lifted yourself by pressing down with the foot. This is important because it is the first in a series of energies that have additive value (in the sense of constructive interference) and the accumulation of this energy is the grand ultimate force or fa jin. An error in any one of the accumulative energies results in a loss of power. The direction of the force of the strumming of the yongchuan must be upward toward the emitting hand. If you actively press downward then the arrow of direction, or the direction the energy will move, is downward instead of upward toward hand.

The stored forces of chan sichou should be felt in the ankle, leg, knee and thigh. This is a kinesthetic sensation of the torsion caused by turning the waist. It is a function of the mechanics of twisting muscle and not the contraction of muscle. This makes for a rigid appendage similar to the stiffening of a twisted rope, and because of this stiffening, the strumming is delivered directly to the hip area. This can be tested by rotating the waist and then strumming the yongchuan. The energy should be translated into a lifting and rotation of the hip area. Practice with this should fine-tune this portion of the fa jin cycle. This element of the fa jin sequence must be coordinated with the breath. This is the yang portion of fa jin in which the energy is actively constituted and distributed to the fingertips. It is not merely a coordination of the cycle and the breath, but instead it is a following of the breath. Exhalation is soft and flowing, in which the breath and the pulse caused by the strumming are delivered simultaneously, where the breath is the device used to coordinate the activity. It must feel as if the breath is clearing a path for the flow of this pulse of qi. The visualization is essential from several standpoints; first, visualization in and of itself can encourage the access needed to the realm of po, second, the smooth gentle breathing encourages song which is needed to allow the free flow of qi; and third, by placing the attention on various parts of the body, those minute changes such as the nine pearls and beautiful lady's hand, yu nu shou, are facilitated.

The transition from the hip joint through the hui yin can be difficult. It is at this point that the chan sichou created by the turning of the waist begins to unwind, and causes the reverse rotation of the waist, and the energy must then be pushed through this area with the breath in combination with the compression of the qi belt and the sacral pump. The direction of the breath is reversed from inhaling to exhaling at the time of the strumming (note that this is true only for ming jing and an jing). It is downward at the front of the abdomen on the inhale and the qi ball is rotated allowing the energy of the breath to then move upward and push through the hui yin. Effort must be made to push the pulse of energy through the hui yin point because of the natural constrictions in this area.

From the sacral pump, the pulse moves along the spine carried by moving contractions of the intercostal muscles and the muscle attachments at the rib spine attachment points. The exhale is a limited, controlled release of the breath as a push upward to the ming men point where it is completely released in conjunction with the forward thrust of the yu nu shou. This forward thrust of the yu nu shou is not a separate movement of the hand and arm, but must be a result of the waist pulling the arm and hand forward by the turning of the waist. If it is not done in this manner then the nine pearls have lost their integrity and the pathway for the qi is broken. Whole body power must exist for the entire length of the qi movement from foot to hand in order to gain the explosive power of fa jin.

In order to move the striking hand forward, it is necessary to transfer the energy from the rear foot to the forward foot and then bounce this force upward. This is done in a manner that keeps the spinal axis upright, just as a juggler balances a pole on his hand. This also allows the head to remain on the same plane and move smoothly assisting in orientation.

6-7 An Jing

The difference between an jing (push force) and fa jin (striking force) is a subtle but important one. Contact is made with the body of the opponent with either one or two hands or with the palms in direct contact with the body with an jing. This is a limiting factor in the rotation of the waist and eliminates the power derived from the yu nu shou. In order to compensate for this loss, it is necessary to exert a force in the opposite direction of the push from the back of the hand to the center of the Taiji practitioner. To make this more obvious, pretend you are holding a ball against the chest and compressing it inward toward your center. Now hold that posture and rotate the palm outward while maintaining the compression of the ball. Release in the compression of the ball yields a forward movement of the hand that was compressing the ball. This is in keeping with the classical expression "if you wish to go right you must first go left," therefore if you wish to press or push forward, you must first exert a force in the opposite direction.

An jing differs also with respect to the nature of the force generated. Just prior to the complete expulsion of air from the lungs, the waist is over rotated or compressed into the rear foot to store power for use in the form of old ox power or jiu gongniu jing. The waist is first stored to the left and then over rotated to the right so that the push is from the left foot and delivered to the right hand with a final counter rotation of the waist to the left. This is a double rotation of the waist, and old ox power occurs in both, but it is pre-eminent in an jing. In fa jin it occurs as a shallow arc in the opposite direction before the beginning of the initial rotation of the waist.

6-8 The Bubbling Well

The bubbling well or yongchuan is located mid point on the ball of the foot. It is important that the strumming of the bubbling well be from a strong root. Grasping the ground with the toes is an aid in developing this strong root, and it moves the center of effort back onto the yongchuan point. This has the effect of relieving the strain of the thrust on the ligaments supporting the toes. Constant use and excessive force derived from fa jin can result in tendinitis or cramping if the center of effort is not moved back to the yongchuan point.

The yongchuan is the endpoint of the kidney meridian, which is, involved in general health in the Chinese qi gong system. This means that every time you press the yongchuan while practicing at the lazhu then you are stimulating this meridian point for healthful benefits.

6-9 The Fascia, Ligaments and Smooth Muscle

The storage of energy within the body in the practice of Taiji is not normally within the large muscle groups, but is instead as in the tantien, stored in the fascia of the abdomen using the inherent elasticity of the fibrous fascia, the muscles of the diaphragm and in other cases the attachments and ligament of the joints and skeletal apparatus. Some of the storage is a result of pneumatic and hydraulic pressures resulting from compression within the body. Particular attention must be made to the storage of energy within the fascia. Energy is normally stored in the fascia, but it is not utilized in a conventional sense in the martial arena. Energy storage occurs because of the natural elasticity of the fascia in the same manner as a rubber band can store energy.

6-10 The Tantien

The tantien is located about two fingers below the navel and about three fingers inward. It is located near the geometric center of the body. The geometric center of a square or rectangle, for instance, is the juncture point of the two diagonals drawn from each corner to the opposite corner. The juncture of all these diagonals on the geometric shape of the human body would theoretically be the geometric center of that body. Conceptually this is important because if the geometric center and the actual center of mass are in vertical alignment, then the object will not topple. This is one of the primary reasons why the attention is centered on the tantien. All movement in a martial perspective is like that of a spider in which all movement was made as if it originated from this central body. All expanding and contracting movements originate from there.

There is another reason there is a martial interest in the tantien, perhaps more important than the geometric center, this involves the energy system of the body. The tantien serves as a reservoir of energy which can be drawn on for various martial purposes. There is mechanical storage here that facilitates fa jin, but there is also a storage of qi in this area which is a deliberate accumulation of this ethereal energy. The deliberate circulation of qi by the small universe circulation or other qi gong methods results in a storage of qi in this area. It is important that qi be available on a seconds notice or the results could be disastrous. This area contains an enormous amount of fascia and smooth muscle that would allow storage of qi.

6-11 Raise the Shoulders and Hollow the Chest

This is a very subtle means of storing energy within the posture and can produce a remarkable supplement to the forces of fa jin and an jing. The classics tell you to do this, but they do not specify the reasons or conditions under which this practice should be performed. The effect of this is very similar to the sine wave of a snapped whip in which the wave front accelerates as it approaches the rigid tip. This accelerated pulse within the human body is created by the forward thrust of the hips in fa jin and an jing combined with the straightening of the spine. This is exactly what occurs with the rounding of the arms in the push portion of the form and the straightening of the arms with the forward thrust of the hips. At the same time as the arms are straightened, the previously raised shoulders and hollowed chest should be straightened. In fa jin the straightening should also occur with the forward thrust of the hips.

6-12 Opening and Closing

Closing refers to the storage phase of the transfer of energy from the arms across the shoulders and between the shoulders in the peng posture. Opening within old ox power and the peng position are on the emission phase. Opening is the release of energy across the shoulders from the spine to the arms and within both postures; it is on the emission phase. As with other forms of storage and release, the energy must follow the breath, therefore, storing on the inhale and releasing on the exhale. In the internal styles as you advance from ming jing (visible force) to an jing (hidden force) and finally to hua jing (perfect force), the breathing and application of force will change from a simple inhale/exhale to an extended inhale with an almost indiscernible exhale. Both ming jing and an jing will exhale on release of the energy of fa jin. This is a perceptual occurrence that follows the normal breathing pattern in using force. The breath, however, in hua jing is an inhale on the opening phase and exhale on the closing phase. This tricks the body into being song on fa jin because this inhale is a normal relaxed state. It also serves to compress the time interval at the release end of the strike. The release itself is a final closing posture in the sequence in the sense of a gentle unforced release. Remember the difference between and explosion and a fire of equal energy is the time interval of the release of energy. The inhale on striking within hua jing contains the energy within the body until the release at the termination of the strike.

6-13 Cracking the Whip

This is a very subtle point and is merely a means of enhancing the effect of the storage and release of energy by the turning of the waist. When you have stored the energy by the rotation of the waist toward the rear foot and the rotation has ended, then before you start the reverse rotation, bounce the energy in the storage direction and then toward the emitting hand to add to the momentum of the forward release. If you visualize the actual cracking of the whip, you will realize the drawing of the whip back is not a passive action but has an active stop to it the accelerates the tip in the storage phase and the forward acceleration is added to this when the backward moving storage is complete The wind up has served as a means of assembling the nine pearls and the chan sichou together, but the second tightening of the compression or rotation serves to put this all together in one controlled pulse of energy.

The handle end of the whip is the beginning of the discharge of energy, and the end of the cycle is the cracking of the whip, which results when the movement of the sine wave is stopped abruptly with the hand. In fa jin, this crack of the whip results when the forward motion is stopped by the forward yongchuan pressing on the ground. This is the same as the abrupt stoppage of the handle of a whip.

It should be noted that the cracking of the whip is found in ming jing and an jing and not within the expression of hua jing. The abrupt stop of an jing and ming jing is missing. This is accomplished by extending the inhale from the storage phase through the emission phase with only short soft unforced exhalation at the point of contact. In practice at the candle, the absence of the rebound from the crack of the whip is quite noticeable. It is one of the evident signs that you are in fact acquiring hua jing.

6-14 Releasing the Qi

The energy of fa jin must be released completely or it will rebound back into the body and release itself in one of the nine pearls that is no longer in firm connection. There is a directional component to the release of qi that is important in eliminating this rebound of energy. If the release is linear, it must be understood that the rebound is in the reverse direction. With a direct linear strike, the hand, arm and shoulder are in alignment. This means that it serves as a direct conduit for the return energy, and it will follow this pathway to the first unconnected pearl and release energy there.

By rounding the structure such as in the beautiful lady's hand, the rebound is dissipated at an angle to the direct alignment, which diverts the energy into empty space. If a straight linear strike is necessary, then the release itself must be rounded or circular. The release or stoppage of the fist is done in a circular manner so that the release is either on the upward or downward segment of the circle. This can be a large circle or an imperceptible circle, as long as the circle of release is not in the same plane as the extended arm. The rebound must be into empty space. In other words, the axis of rotation must not be the limb itself, but perpendicular or some other angle to it.

6-15 The Six Circular Accelerations

The six circular accelerations is a look at the underlying dynamics of the forces within fa jin and an jing from an angular momentum concept to get some perspective on the forces generated and how they interact. In each case, the motions are an arc of a much larger circle with the striking arm as the radius and in some instances a portion of the spine as the radius. The first circle is a result of the turning of the waist and the momentum gained by moving a distance off from the center; this is further increased by moving the fist out onto a longer radius at the end of the cycle. The effect is much like the movement of hands in ice-skating. The skater extends the hands outward to slow down the rotating body and brings them inward to accelerate the body. The martial interest is the acceleration of the hand, which is the reverse of the skater's interest. As we accelerate the waist in a constant manner, we gain acceleration of the fist by moving it farther out on the radius of the circle. This is the second acceleration. Even though the period of rotation is the same at each radius, the distance covered is greater on the outer circle.

The third acceleration is within the beautiful lady's hand, which is a graceful curvature of the hand forming an arc of a given radius, and by changing the curvature to one of a longer radius; we gain additional acceleration. The fourth acceleration is merely the angular momentum derived from the radius with its center at the heel of the rear foot and the arc formed by the hips in a forward thrust. This thrust is an arc that moves the vertical spine forward.

The fifth acceleration is a sine wave, which is also a circular function that is contained in the classical teachings of "raise the shoulders and hollow the chest."

When straightening occurs, this sine wave translates the energy in the manner of a whip sending the force up the spine and then out the forward arm to the hand. This results in the same acceleration as that at the stiff end of the whip due to the inverse relationship between amplitude of the wave and the velocity.

The sixth acceleration is that of opening and closing, and in the same manner that the beautiful lady's hand results in an acceleration caused by increasing the curvature of the arc, so does this cause a similar acceleration.

6-16 Compressing the Spring

It helps to think of the storage of energy from the turning of the waist and the strumming of the yongchuan as the compression of a spring. The first compression is from the turning of the waist to compress the energy into the foot and connect the nine pearls, there is a second compression, which involves the further compression of the spring from both ends. This is as if you had the spring in your hands and compressed it inward with both hands and then bounced it inward one more time without releasing the first compression. The purpose of the first compression is to get all body alignments and connections made. This makes the final compression correct and therefore effective.

6-17 The Taiji Ready Stance

The Taiji ready stance, which is grasp the sparrow's tail with the forward toe raised, is unique to Taiji. The purpose of this unusual, ungainly and unimpressive stance, is that it forces the hip over the heel of the rear leg, and in doing this it forces the balance to be on that one point, in alignment with the with the rear leg which is the ideal stance for fa jin. Much that appears awkward and unusual in Taiji is for the purposes of generating the energy of fajin or the delivery of this energy into the opponent.

6-18 The Nine Pearls

To gain insight into the essence of the nine pearls, make use a long piece of rope or a martial arts belt. Stand on one end of the strap and grasp the other end in such a manner that the strap is tight across the buttocks waist and back. When you turn your waist, you will notice that it is articulated into a movement that is transferred all the way from your rear foot to your forward upward extended hand. This connection is essential to creating fa jin. It is the basis upon which all the accumulative forces of fa jin are derived. It is the channel for the free flow of qi and the impulse generated by the strumming of the yongchuan. This is a two-way passage of energy. This connection must be made on the inward flow and storage of qi and it must be sustained on the emission stage. It is helpful to practice with the strap across the back in order to gain a feel for this connection. Fa jin will not occur even if you have everything else in place and there is no continuity within the nine pearls. This has a very noticeable sensation to it if it is correctly done. The movement of the pulse across the back area is something that has to be cultivated and this is done by attending to these sensations.

6-19 Drawing in the Energy from the Hands

Just as the energy of tumo of the Tibetans or ri qi of the Chinese is delivered to the hands from the xin (heart), so too can the energy be reversed and delivered from the hands for storage internally. The energy drawn inward should be visualized as a thin cool stream of air. Its movement should be visualized as coming from the hands to the heels. This relates to the Chinese expression "an immortal breathes through his heels." An immortal to the Chinese is one who has experienced enlightenment, and the expression of one who breathes through his heels is in reference to the practice of qi gong in which the individual visualizes the energy flowing to and from the feet in the Zhan Zhuang exercise. Qi gong is considered along with martial arts and meditation, to be a pathway to enlightenment.

6-20 The Perceptual Difference between Qi and Fa jin

Fa jin is the storage of energy kinetically within the body by various means and the release of this energy in fa jin can be seen at the candle visually as a rebounding of energy at the hands. This snap back of a pulse of energy is characteristic of the release of fa jin. There is a noticeable difference between the qualitative release of qi and fa jin. The release of qi as opposed to fa jin is simply a flowing from the movement and is generally accompanied by surprise on the part of the practitioner because nothing happened at the hand end of the emission. There was no rebound of the hand in the release of the energy that is so characteristic of fa jin. There was no feeling of contraction or compression that usually accompanies fa jin. All that can be felt is the soft fluid movement of the hand as it displaces air and there is the barest sensation of something fluid moving through the arms and hand, but there is nothing of the force and energy consistent with fa jin. Fa jin is mechanical in its development, delivery and release. Qi, however, is ephemeral and produces great power with seemingly little effort, and with an almost nonexistent kinesthetic sensation.

The difference in the ability to produce the extinguishing of the candle flame at a distance is also remarkably different. The ability to put the flame out with fa jin drops off rapidly after twelve inches and is almost impossible beyond eighteen inches. To extinguish the candle flame beyond eighteen inches, it is necessary to use qi (hua jing) or at the very least, fa jin with qi enhancement. This is a smooth flow of energy that is derived out of the fluid movements of the body preceded by the visualization of the movements by the mind of the practitioner. The energy developed is a continuum extending from the visible force of ming jing and hidden force of an jing on through the perfect force hua jing. All forces along this continuum have a qi component, which becomes manifest as you progress along this continuum. It is the nature of hua jing that the higher the qi element, then the more trance like the state of po becomes. The truly bizarre things that are expressed about Taiji are from this elevated state of existence. The farther from the wisdom mind, then the more powerful the force becomes and at the same time it becomes more difficult to initiate because of this distance from the controlling aspects of the yi mind.

6-21 The Relationship between Emitted and Borrowed Energy

The connections made in fa jin for the nine pearls and the visualizations before the candle are the same as those for borrowing jing, except that the direction of movement of the energy is in reverse. If you understand the idea that in training for fa jin, you are also training for all the other techniques requiring a connection and pathway for the emission of qi then you will progress rapidly.

6-22 San guanxi

The three connections or san guanxi are guide posts that assist you in making the correct hand foot and body positions that will facilitate in creating whole body power and fa jin (see figure 7).

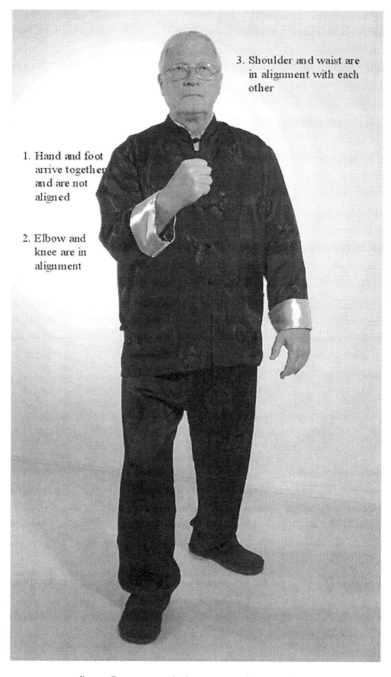

3. Shoulder and waist are
   in alignment with each
   other

1. Hand and foot
   arrive together
   and are not
   aligned

2. Elbow and
   knee are in
   alignment

figure 7. san guanxi, three external connections

The three external san guanxi are; hand and foot, elbow and knee, hips and waist. The hand and foot connection is the idea that both must arrive at the same time. In order for there to be whole body power, the body must move as a unit in a predetermined manner. To ensure that the hand is in contact with the opponent when the energy arrives, it is necessary to coordinate the sequence of the separate parts. The hand and foot coordination should be trained in such a way that the arrival of the pulse of energy is of primary concern. This can be trained at the candle by a mock intercepting motion with the striking hand, while in a cat stance, then a half step backward and then stepping forward to fa jin at the candle, while you place your attention on the connection between hand and foot. The position of the hand is at your location of maximum strength. This is done without placing your attention on the hand. When we place our attention on something, it is with the wisdom mind. We want to cultivate po the ancient mind in any simulated usage of power.

The second of the three connections is the elbow and the knee. This is not a readily discernable connection unless you try it. The first and most important thing you will notice is that it forces your hand to move onto your centerline. There is a tendency, when doing the hand and foot connection, to place the hand in line with the forward foot. This is incorrect. The hand should be relaxed, as in the jade lady's hand and by coordinating the elbow with the knee, the hand will effortlessly remain on the center. You are always admonished to keep your hand on your center because it is from this position that you most effectively deliver the forces derived from fa jin. This is a means of training you to properly move and be certain that when the energy pulse arrives the energy is being delivered from your most powerful position. The unusual look of movements within Taiji is because of this need to maintain the center when moving so there is no loss of energy.

The third and final external connection (there are also three internal connections) is the hips and waist. As you stand before the candle with hips and waist in alignment so that your body is in perfect forward alignment and the hand and foot and the elbow and knee connections are made, fa jin can occur effortlessly. When you rotate for an intercept, all of these connections must also be maintained. If for instance, you rotate your waist and not your hips, then your hand will move off your centerline and will be in line with your side. These alignments are critical for the delivery of the impulse of qi as it is released from the yongchuan.

The real secret to the external san guanxi lies in the fact that the three connections force your hand onto the centerline of your body and force a coordinated movement without your attention centering on your hand. Your attention is elsewhere, on the alignments of the three connections. If you were to place your attention on your hand and attempt to keep it on your center, you would ultimately be using force against force because your attention is there and it is the wisdom mind that is predominant. This centers your hand and places your attention away from your hand and any effort to express force.

The three internal connections are; mind and intent; qi and force; and posture and bones. The external san guanxi must be acquired and properly used before the internal san guanxi can be instituted. Mind and intent are entwined within the intricate the patterns of wu-wei, song and yi yi yin qi. It is a balancing act in which you must be song, at the same time you must act without doing, and you must be within the domain of po. It is only then that you can lead the qi with the yi mind. This is only possible when the yi mind and po are in close proximity and a balance has been reached between the mind and body, or the hun (human aspects) and the po or (animal aspects) are in harmony.

Qi can be defined as energy and force can be defined as the movement of mass over a distance. Certainly, it is much more complicated, but for our purposes, this simple distinction can be made. In the Chinese martial arts, force i.e. muscular force would be called li. The external styles place heavy emphasis on the use of li. The connection between qi and force li is that within Taiji and other internal arts, the use of li is minimized and the use of qi is maximized. Muscular force is used only where necessary in maintaining balance and the minimal movement of body mass.

The connections between posture and bones are not a complicated, yet they can be very confusing. The bones of the spine and all other structures from foot to head must be aligned one over the other so that there is no leaning and no undue stress placed on the skeletal structure that will cause muscular stress. The ming men must be straightened by tilting the hips forward and the chin must be pushed backward to straighten the spine at the neck. The head is kept in line with the spine by a slight upward pressure that creates a feeling of lightness as if the head were suspended by a thread. The feet move nimbly to maintain a balance under the straight rod of the spine. All structures must be in line as a means of support without stressing the muscles or creating unnecessary tension. Movements must be light and lively. The primary principle of san guanxi is that the center of attention is placed away from the point of effort so that it is done in a mindless and unconcerned manner i.e. within the realm of po.

7

Whole Body Power

7-1 Components of Zhen Jing

Zhen jing is whole body power. This concept is consistent with moving the body as an integrated unit, not as a rigidly anchored one piece but as a coordination of separate pieces. It consists of being centered, therefore keeping your mind on the tantien (yi shou tantien) and moving as if all effort originated from this center. It also includes maintaining the center, which requires you to keep your hands on the centerline at a distance no farther than your center of power. The center of power can be determined by drawing a line along the shin of the rear leg and following this line as it intersects your hand (see figure 8). The forward hand should be on this intersection point of the centerline and this line drawn from the shin. This is your most powerful position or location for the forward hand.

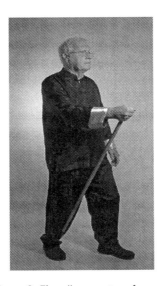

figure 8. Zhen jing, center of power

All postures and striking methods must be made in with this point in mind. The hand must always be on the centerline as you move from one position to another, as much as possible and it should be as close to the center of power as possible. When moving the feet do not move the feet first and then the hand, the waist should guide movement of both in a coordinated manner. If you move your hand by using the shoulder muscles, then you are using the body as a rigid and separate stationery frame in which your hand is moved off center away from your center of power thus making you more vulnerable to attack.

In order to deliver the forces of whole body power from the feet to the hand through the nine pearls, each nine pearl must be connected, which then transforms this energy pulse into a martial force. It then is possible to thread the qi through the nine pearls and deliver it to the hand. The only difference between an jing, fa jin and zhen jing is that the body is in motion in zhen jing and you are carrying the qi along with you in that motion so that you can deliver it in a coordinated manner into the body of the opponent through some technique. It then becomes necessary to learn how to carry this stored qi along with you as you move into position for a technique, and then to be able to transfer this learning into the practice of the form, so that you can carry the qi along as you move through the form. One of the principle differences in the forms of delivery of the energy is the focus or intent of the delivery. An jing is a directional force applied to move the opponent, fa jin is a concentration of energy that is delivered to an organ or vital point or the meridians and channels of the energy system, while zhen jing is the coordinated movement from the center that manipulates the opponent rather than delivering a force directly into him. If For instance in a grab right hand to right hand, the coordinated movement of the waist with the hand remaining on center, nine pearls intact and the effective movement of qi from the feet results in an irresistible force pulling the opponent forward into an unbalanced position with little effort. All of those postural requirements that apply to Taiji are a prerequisite for the implementation of zhen jing. The hips should be tilted slightly forward to close the ming men; chin pushed slightly in to straighten spine; knees slightly bent; breathe from the tantien, and press the tongue against the teeth.

All coordinated movement should be guided by the breath, which is moved by the tantien (Buddhist or reverse Taoist breathing) and not the intercostal muscles of the chest. Stepping is coordinated, the forward foot is placed on the ground heel first, and then the center of balance is moved to the forward foot. This is emphasized, because it is more important that you do not lose your balance than it is for the technique to succeed. Most martial arts use gravity in concert with stepping as a force to manipulate the opponent. This leaves the adept vulnerable during the natural occurring free fall so that the he can be caught in the midst of floating and easily dispatched. Floating is defined as that part of stepping sequence in which the opponent is compelled to finish the step in the free fall portion of it in order to maintain his balance. His balance has then been moved forward and it cannot be recovered. In Taiji, the balance is never sacrificed for the technique. If there is no balance first, then there is no technique. Whole body power consists of moving the body in an integrated and coordinated manner from a stable base. If this stable base is not there, then there is no whole body power. Gravity is only used after the placement of the moving foot has occurred and stability is assured. Taiji is not falling into a stance. Each move is deliberate, balanced and coordinated.

7-2 Borrowing Energy from the Opponent

It is during the storage phase of the fa jin or an jing cycle that the borrowing of energy will occur. The directional arrow indicating the flow of energy is toward the feet in this phase, and in Taiji, the initial movement is predominantly a defensive one. The energies for fa jin and an jing are complex and constructively additive. These energies are amassed and then expand into an explosive force. Borrowing energy from the opponent is a supplement to this aggregate of energies. The channels used to store energy for an jing and fa jin are the same as those used to generate borrowed energy. Practice in storing energy for the hard jings is a practice for borrowing energy. Jie jing or borrowing energy is not adding energy to the opponents own energy, but is instead the return of the energy he has delivered to you, by bouncing this energy off the yongchuan and delivering it back in the same strength he delivered it. If it was a soft jing then that is what is returned. If, instead, it was a hard jing, then what is returned is the same energy and he receives back what he has aggressively sent to harm you. This is a difficult technique to master, but it is a high level of attainment and is effective in neutralizing an aggressive opponent.

To learn jie jing, it necessary to concentrate on the storage phases of lazhu fangfa, and use the candle method to visualize the storage and return of the opponent's energy.

7-3 Moving the Body as a Unit

Taiji is the study of storing energy within the body and moving while reserving this energy pulse and then having the capacity to emit this energy effortlessly into the opponent. To accomplish this and effortlessly utilize the forces of Taiji, move the body as one complete unit, not as a rigid structure, but as one in which it is moved as a coordinated and integrated whole. This movement is coordinated with the flow of the breath with the idea that it is one movement. The sensations derived from each aspect of the movement are kinesthetic in nature and each has its own particular quality or feeling. It is important to train these sensations separately and internalize them. The integration of these sensations into one complete whole is essential. The yi mind does this since po has no feedback from the kinesthetic sensory system. The feel of the coordinated nine pearls is distinctive from the rigid force of the external styles. There is relaxation except at the points of connection that are the nine pearls. The coordination of hand and foot movements is necessary so that they arrive at the proper moment. Turn the waist with the hand on the centerline of the body. Vertically align the spine with no leaning in any direction. Move the upright spine as a juggler moves under a long staff to balance it on his hand, maintaining the vertical alignment of the center of effort, the tantien with the center gravity. The energy follows the breath in a coordinated manner, from the upward lift of the yongchuan: through the nine pearls; through the turning of the waist; up the spine and out to the fingertips such that it arrives when your hand arrives at the target.

The motion of the body as a unit is an unnatural movement. Train this with due diligence. One of the most successful ways of training the movement of the body as a whole is lazhu fangfa. It works because there is feed back from the candle to tell you when this is successful.

7-4 Connecting the Various Parts

Moving the body as one coordinated unit of mass does not guarantee the movement of qi in coordination with this singular movement. The qi must be pushed to the end of all the hairs is a common expression of Taiji. This is true of ming jing and an jing but not of hua jing. Hua jing is what distinguishes other styles from Taiji. Many train in a low level of hua jing, but it is Taiji that excels in this and all training, especially whole body power is trained with this in mind as it is the essence of Taiji. It is this active push of the qi in the lower levels of training that must be coordinated with the breath. It is a slow methodical pushing of the qi up through all the pathways provided by the nine pearls that this connection occurs. When the classics say that an immortal is one who breathes through his heels, it means that it is one who practices qi gong. It is qi gong practiced in a specific way. The cultivation of the nine pearls is by way of qi gong practice. Each individual pearl is acquired by long practice in Zhang Zhuang, where you actively test each connection to see if it is connected, and through visualization the energy is perceived to move from the hand to the yongchuan in the storage phase and then from yongchuan to the hand in the emission phase. These visualizations train the mind to lead the qi or place it in the body wherever it is appropriate. These visualizations are one of placing the mind on the energy pulse as you feel it move through the body and at the same time that you assist this movement. Remember that mental activity always has a physical component to it, no matter how small, and in this instance, it will grow with use and serve to move the pulse along. The push is probably a result of training the vascular system to constrict and the contraction of the tendons and smooth muscles along the pathways. By actively visualizing this pulse moving through the body, you are building a trained sequence that will improve with the visualizations. The specifics of the contractions are not important. It is only important that you cultivate this feeling of a pulse moving through the body. It is this pulse that connects the various parts on the inhale, as if you were drawing in energy with the breath and making these connections as you store the energy, for later delivery of the pulse back along the same pathway. It is a two-pronged approach. It is more important to learn to make the connections on the inhale than it is on the exhale when doing an jing and ming jing. There is no energy if there is no storage of it on the inhale. No matter how good your fa jin, there is no energy with out this storage phase.

To assist in moving the body as a unit, it is necessary to keep san guanxi uppermost in the mind and train it until it is internalized. San guanxi is a means of coordinating movement by attending to three external and three internal connections. The external three connections are relevant for zhen jing. The three external connections are, hand and foot, knee and elbow, waist and hips. If you pay close attention to this, you will realize that if the hand is kept on the center and in approximate vertical alignment with the foot, they will arrive at the same time. The elbow and the knee in alignment will result in the hand remaining on the centerline of the body. If the waist and hips are connected then the body will be aligned to enhance zhen jing.

7-5 The Practice of the Form as a Practice of Zhen Jing

Each posture within the form has its own unique way of storing, carrying forward and releasing energy. The intermediate position of holding the ball is a means of storing energy. The energy derived from compressing the ball by inward compression of the hands is the same as the inward compression of the ball in the peng stance. The beautiful lady's hand, yu nu shou, is a means of storing energy within the graceful curves of the arm and hand. The curvature of the arms and hands in the push section of the sequence grasp the sparrow's tail powers the extremities as they move in the storage phase as if rolling them over a ball. Raising the shoulders and hollowing the chest in the same sequence results in the release of energy stored in this posture in the form of a sine wave, which when straightened is comparable to the snap of a whip. Much of the uniqueness of the look of the Taiji form is the storage, carrying forward and release of energy within the Taiji form. Chinese martial artists refer to an individual who exhibits a showy martial technique with no power as one who has "flowery fists and brocade legs." The appearance of power, which you display in doing the form, comes from incorporating zhen jing in the practice of the Taiji form. An experienced practitioner of Taiji can tell, by your ability to express whole body power in the form, at what level of Taiji you are performing.

7-6 Moving the Qi

The postures are precise in their expression so that they do not hinder the free flow of qi. The many corrections in posture that the student suffers are so that there are no defects or blockages to this free flow of qi. To move the qi from the yongchuan to the hand, store and carry the qi through the movement without it blocking it or by dissipating it within the form. This is the single most important feature of whole body power. It is in moving the body as a coordinated unit that fa jin and an jing are produced. The body as a coiled spring releases energy at the proper time, and the energy that flows through this uncoiling and eventual release emits the force at the extreme end of the cycle.

Refining this mechanical pulse through years of practice creates the real force of qi. It is in training for these specific forces that conditions are set up for the flow of qi. The analogy of the stick drawing a furrow from a puddle and creating a pathway for the flow of water is a good one. Many take the energies of fa jin derived at this stage as the end point of the force curve. It is only the beginning. It is by refining fa jin that we develop the true power inherent in Taiji, which is hua jing. This refining is done over years of practice with a powerful fa jin in which you attempt to reduce the usage of muscles, movement, and the use of kinetic forces in generating the explosive power, and eventually convert it into a soft pliable energy that works over longer distances. The effective range of fa jin is about six to twelve inches to extinguish the candle. To go beyond this requires the application of qi in its pure form. It is, however, necessary to first learn to properly and effectively use fa jin. This is for martial and protective purposes and as a means of developing the pathways. Lazhu fangfa develops and fosters the pathways that lead to fa jin.

7-7 The Sine Wave of Power

A sine wave is mathematically a circular function, and this is what we do in Taiji. We move in circles, big circles and small circles and describe circular movements with our hands, feet, and body in a non-ending flow of storing and emitting energy. The sine wave represents the yin and yang of Taoist philosophy in which at its maximum you return to its minimum. Each posture represents the storage of energy within this circular function. This graceful arc (a circular segment) stores energy. It is the sine wave formed by the raising of the shoulders and hollowing of the chest that stores energy. It is the curvature of the hands and arms of the storage phase of push in grasp the sparrow's tail and its flow from positive to negative form that generates the push.

A sine wave is a circle function graphically represented over time that moves continuously by forming, ending and reforming along the continuum of time. This is the form of Taiji. It flows like the sine wave and the real power of Taiji is not the force of fa jin, but the fact that it does not stop and continually flows on like the "Great River" and continually presses forward, advancing on you with the ebb and flow of an irresistible force until you succumb.

7-8 Components of Whole Body Power

Dividing whole body power into the storage phase and the emission phase allows us to distinguish between entering and emitting force. The storage phase within this sequence is as follows. The extremity that is the source of fajin initiates the storage phase. If you are to emit fa jin with the hand, then you would begin storage from that extremity by visualizing the energy moving inward from the hand to the foot. It is along this pathway that the energy will return in a magnified form. Connection of the nine pearls occurs as the visualization process progresses through each segment of the pathway and these connections yield a specific kinesthetic feel at each pearl. Constant attention to the nine pearls in the qi gong exercise Zhan Zhuang develops a kinesthetic feeling. Maintain the hand on the centerline at a distance of maximum power. The hand moves with the turning of the waist not by separate muscular control, and does not deviate from this position until aligned with the center of the opponent. It then moves directly to the target on the centerline through the coordinated movement of the body, not by the separate movement of the hand and arm.

Rotating the waist toward the rear foot results in a torque and compression of the long muscles of the leg and thigh, and this is the storage of chan sichou or silk reeling. Raising the shoulders and hollowing creates a sine wave like curvature to the spine that stores the energy within this curve. Raise the front foot so that it is in a "cat stance" or elevate the front toes so that only the heel is resting on the ground. This shifts the balance over the rear leg and it results in maintaining the one point of the Taiji sphere.

The breathing on inhale is the guiding factor for the visualization of the inward draw of energy. Draw the breath in slowly and effortlessly as a soft, thin cool stream of air. The diaphragm should be used to draw in this breath, note that drawing in the breath is accomplished with the intercostal muscles of the chest relaxed to avoid tension in this area. The abdominal area should be visualized as a downward movement to the front, which corresponds to the turning of the qi ball.

To begin the second phase, which is the emitting stage of this cycle of whole body power, it is necessary to further compress into the chan sichou and by a further compression of the yongchuan by rotating in the same direction as the initial turning of the waist (toward the rear foot). This serves to create a bounce, which will serve as a signal to press the yongchuan in an upward lifting manner, which activates the turning of the waist toward the forward foot. At this stage, it is necessary to curl the toes to move the point of contact with the floor to the yongchuan point. This bounce is also the signal for the slow exhale of breath (ming jing and an jing only) which should be a thin cool stream of air. The effort exerted to move the pulse forward is not a muscular one, but is instead a push, that is upward and along the channel that was prescribed by the inward storage of energy. This is distinctly different from the effort of external styles, and this has an internal feel of contraction of the bones along this pathway and not one of the contractions of external muscles. It is this pulse that is being pushed forward in conjunction with the coordinated movement of the body. This visualization of the movement of this pulse must be cultivated and reinforced by practice to keep it foremost in the emission cycle. The push is critical to proper performance. It should be understood as a minute squeezing or compression of tissues; particularly those of the sacrum; intercostal muscles; and those long muscles at the spinal column that moves the pulse in a manner in which it appears to squeeze the pulse forward as though it were a section of toothpaste.

7-9 Using the Bows of Posture in Zhen Jing

The first bow becomes the beautiful lady's hand or yu nu shou. The rounded aspects of this bow are a means of storage, and by the straightening of these, it yields the release of opposing forces, which is similar to the effects of a compressed automotive spring. It is rounded in appearance during storage and has the appearance of a recurved bow in release.

The second bow is formed by the arc that begins at the heel of the back foot and progresses upward through the hip along the back through the ming men and jade pillow until it reaches the top of the head (bai hui). This bow is activated by the rotation of the waist. The bow is drawn by the rotation of the waist into the direction of the rear foot. It is released and rotated away from the rear foot.

The third bow contains the arch formed by the legs. It extends from the rear heel up the rear leg through the hui yin and terminates in the forward heel. The third bow is activated by the forward thrust of the hips while maintaining an erect spine.

7-10 Rippling the Spine in the Third Bow

Raising the Shoulders and hollowing the chest are a means of storing and releasing energy that occur in the second bow in the storage phase and are released within the third bow. This is an additive force that tends to accumulate energy and supplement the sine wave of pulse that is delivered to the hand in fa jin. It is very much like the way a snake strikes by curving its back and then removing the curves with muscular contraction.

7-11 To Move Right You Must First Move Left

Whole body power emanates from the internal storage of energy within the body. If the technique is to go in one direction, then in order to store the energy of whole body power, it is necessary to first move in the opposite direction. There is an additional benefit from this movement in the opposite direction. It is the contribution the opponent adds to the equation. If you apply energy in one direction, the opponent will apply an opposing resistance in the opposite direction. The storage phase then has the function of setting the opponent up for movement in the direction you wish because he will resist you in the direction opposite to your real intention.

7-12 Strength of Emitted Pulse

The strength of whole body power can be directly tied to three factors. They are first, the strength of the visualization, second, the strength of the reverse Taoist breath during the storage phase and thirdly, on the emission phase the strength of whole body power is dependent on the outward push of the force to the ends of all the hairs except in hua jing which is a special case to be dealt with later.

7-13 Sensing the Movement of Qi in the Opponent

It is difficult to demonstrate the sensation of energy movement through the body when it occurs with extreme force as in fa jin or even an jing. A simple demonstration using grasping techniques can give the novice an understanding of some of the differences in the movement of qi. The difference to be demonstrated is simply the direction of the flow of qi. If you can control the direction of the flow of qi with no more than a simple change in the grasp of the opponent, then the perception of the direction of flow of qi can be better understood.

If the opponent grasps your left wrist with his right hand, and you are both evenly centered, it is a situation of strength against strength with the opponent in control because of his hand on top of yours. The conflict is evident in the feel of stagnation in the flow of qi. A simple change in grip will alter this situation. If instead of grasping the wrist, the opponent places his ring finger in the joint of the wrist with small finger controlling the movement of the hand in the grasp, the direction of flow of qi has been altered. This can be demonstrated to be a distinct advantage to the opponent. He now controls the direction of flow of the qi. This can be demonstrated by competitively pushing against each other. In this situation it is not difficult for the opponent to move you. There is a demonstrable change in the sensation of flow of qi.

It is possible to alter this flow of qi as demonstrated. Instead of allowing the opponent to grasp you in a martial way that will allow him to control the flow of qi, you move your hand slightly forward before he has grasped you so that his grasp is not with the ring finger in the joint, but is instead upward slightly on the wrist so that it is on the forearm just off the wrist, then the energy flow is reversed and you have the upper hand. The qi will flow in the direction of the opponent and he will be moved.

This is a simple demonstration that will give you the feel of the movement of qi. It will also illustrates that a slight variation in the technique can do immense things to alter who controls the situation, and that it is not necessarily strength that prevails in a direct confrontation.

Section Three:
Hard Jings Training

8

Lazhu fangfa

8-1 Principles of Lazhu fangfa

Lazhu fangfa is the usage of a candle (lazhu) for the purposes of training in the development of fa jin. Its usage extends to the development of borrowing jing or the receiving and neutralizing of energy delivered by the opponent. This is possible because the pathways for storage and emission are the same, and training in the development of one direction effects the performance in the other direction.

Lazhu fangfa is more of an intellectual exercise in that it is training the mind to comprehend the energy as it is moving through the body, so that this energy can be detected and the pathways connected at all points. It is by training the mind that we alter the normal tendency to use muscular force in offensive moves. The mind leads the energy through its pathways in the storage phase and the emission phase. Training the mind is the first principle of lazhu fangfa.

The second principle is: the usage of visualizations as a means of training the mind to coordinate the Taiji form into one integrated whole; including the addition of the fighting sequence training; interception training; and the striking force training. The potential for lethal strikes in fa jin precludes one from actually using it in a fighting sequence as training, therefore visualization is a necessary factor in forming the continuity of the technique and the emission of force. These visualizations are also a means of accessing po, which will be discussed in detail in section four. The visualizations are the glue that binds all these efforts together so that it becomes one complete whole. Each separate function has its own unique training and application, but each in turn must be combined in a manner that does no harm. Visualizations are also an effective tool for training at any time or any place, and are as effective as the actual physical training. It is the mind that is being trained in Taiji, which places great emphasis on visualization training. The physical training is the reduction of effort not the increased usage of external effort. The visualizations tie the separate training together by keying on the opponent as the object of the visualizations. This is the common thread that links them all together. The common opponent within each visualization effort creates this continuity between divergent training methods and comprises the one common factor that links each to the other and makes it one complete whole.

The effect of the candle method is to allow one to use maximum force with minimum effort and still maintain the calm, serene mind that typifies Taiji. One of the most difficult things to overcome is the natural tendency to tense up in threatening or aggressive situations. Working with force at the candle is not the same as a direct confrontation. Even on the mat in a friendly confrontation, it is difficult to get the trainees to relax and not use force. The candle does not have socially significant meanings that would increase tension and overt aggressiveness. It trains in maximum aggressiveness with minimum force. It is a neutral adversary, albeit a tenacious one. It is possible to train oneself in song, which is that relaxed sentience that is so important to Taiji. This calming effect of the candle is the third principle of lazhu fangfa.

The full force of fa jin is not evident unless all the nine pearls are connected properly. Constant practice before the candle with the immediate feedback from it, results in the constant correction of any improperly connected pearl. There is no pathway if the nine pearls are not connected. If there is an improperly connected pearl and the energy rebounds with an incomplete release, then the improperly connected pearl will be the locus of all forces rebounding. For this reason, it is important to train for the nine pearls before maximum power is reached. The connection of the nine pearls is the fourth principle of lazhu fangfa.

The candle is effective for determining just how much power the strike is generating. This can be determined by the wick length, and the distance from the candle that the force is emitted. There are also variations in the consistency of the wax and the candlewick, all of which create conditions for varying the amount of force required to extinguish the candle. One of the factors, which affects the strength of the pulse of energy in fa jin is the degree of storage of energy. This is the fifth principle of lazhu fangfa.

Emitting energy or fa jin is the main function of lazhu fangfa, but it is not the most important. Direct feedback from the candle immediately tells you that the performance is satisfactory or not, but it does not tell you what the cause is. It is only by constant trial and error that all defects can be eliminated. This immediate feedback is the sixth principle of lazhu fangfa.

The seventh principle of lazhu fangfa is using the candle as the opponent. It allows you to determine distance off, and perform a neutralizing technique on an imaginary opponent, which leads direct into a fa jin. This ties the visualization of the interception with the neutralization and then fa jin of the opponent. The imagined opponent is the one thing that makes this training real. Po makes no distinction between real and imagined imagery. If it has all the appropriate emotional and visual signatures that reality has, then essentially, it is real.

The eight principles of lazhu fangfa is that you do not use the central portion of the visual field (fovea) and utilize only the peripheral vision to see the visualization of the opponent and the candle. This assures you that you are training the techniques within po. Initial training, until you become adept at fa jin, will use the fovea. It is in later stages when you can consistently put the candle out that you would begin training in the peripheral visual area.

8-2 Training Methods

Every method of an jing and fa jin that occurs within the Taiji form can be trained before the candle. It is the nature of the form and the desire for a continuous flow of energy from one posture to another that precludes one from releasing fa jin within the form itself. The striking aspects of the form were concealed in the early versions to protect the Yang family when it was required that they teach the form at the emperor's court. This is a tradition that has been carried forward when the Yang style entered the public domain. This does facilitate the development of song while performing the form because there are then no break points in the form, which would stop the free flow of energy.

It is important to duplicate the moves at the candle as they occur in the form so that the strikes at the candle can become integrated with the movements within the form. Visualizations during the performance of the form in reference to the strikes is an additional means of tying the form and lazhu fangfa together into one integrated whole. The training in the form and the candle is reciprocal in that each can reinforce the training of the other, and each in turn can benefit from the training of the other.

It is common practice to have the image of the opponent before you as you do the form. It is also imperative that you have the image of the opponent before you as you work with the candle. It is this imagery of the opponent that ties everything together. This image of the opponent must be cultivated in order to assemble all the separate aspects of training into one concentrated whole.

Taiji is a defensive style martial art, and as such, the first move would be a defensive one. This first move generally is a neutralization of an incoming force in the form of a punch. It is necessary to train this neutralization with visualizations so that it can be integrated within this system of candle strikes. There is no technique in Taiji until there is first contact with the opponent. The first step in any technique of Taiji is to establish contact with the opponent so that with ting jing, you can determine what he is doing, and you do not relinquish contact until he is dispatched or it is imperative because of his efforts that you push him away.

To train in interception and the visualization techniques associated with it requires using a softball, which has the size, shape, and coloration that duplicates that of an average size fist. This is tied with loops of one eighth-inch nylon cord and then hung from a doorway or ceiling so that it swings freely. Interception at first should be with large circles. It should begin with the hands at the side, as they would be in a normal relaxed stance. Most instances of attack are going to come without your being aware that there is a problem or it will be a deliberate deception. The interception should occur at the top of the circle so that the interception occurs when the hand is moving in the same direction as the incoming fist. This results in an imperceptible interception. It more than likely will be imperceptible to you, and you will only be aware of it when you visually discern that your hand is in front of your face with his wrist cradled in the curve of your wrist. When properly done interception techniques occur with out intervention of the yi mind. This means that they occur without feedback and the only aware-ness of the interception is a visual sensing of the captured fist. The techniques to access po should be applied here to escape the meddling ego and they should therefore rely on the more serene and precise po. The interception should begin with the withdrawal of the opponent's fist while it is being chambered for the strike and the interception should ideally arrive in contact with the fist at the beginning of the forward thrust of the opponent's fist. It is possible to arrive before the fist of the opponent is fully chambered and a strike to that fist is possi-ble while it is still moving backward and this can have a devastating effect on the confidence of the attacker, and should send him reeling backward.

Visualizing the opponent chambering his fist should occur prior to swinging the ball outward in preparation for the interception. This visual of the fist being chambered can be practiced in the mirror using a strike with the left fist, which will appear as a right-hand strike in the mirror. Eventually you will be able to visualize without the mirror and with your eyes open. It may only be a limited sense of the attack as visualization, but this will be effective. This must be trained with dedication. There is no defense if there is no interception. The techniques begin when there is contact. If this contact is not under your control, then no technique can be guaranteed to work. This visualization is critical to your defense because it ties the practice of fa jin to the defensive action of interception. Practice at the candle should be integrated within the whole system of lazhu fangfa by accessing po. This is done by using that portion of the visual field (peripheral vision) that is the domain of po. The fovea, that portion of the visual field that is in the center and results in the highly focused vision, is the domain of the yi or wisdom mind. Po has a more immediate response because it is not encumbered by logical, social and emotional considerations. It is not hampered by filtering it through the logical system. Po does not use words and it is primarily visual in its thinking and primal in its understanding. It does not fear death, or more accurately, it does not understand death. In order to understand death it is necessary to have the concepts of past and present. Po operates within the eternal now and has no concept of past and present. By accessing po, our response is immediate and the training methods are not much different except that it is slower, more serene, and it is designed for access to po. The softness of Taiji is every bit as much for access to po as it is for defensive advantages. There is not enough time for the slower reaction of the ego mind during the interception phase. Taiji takes advantage of the longer time for the opponents chambering of the fist, note that this chambering does not occur in fa jin, and every effort must be made to increase this advantage. The ego mind does not operate efficiently in the periphery of vision, which means that if someone were outside the central focused area of vision when they attacked you, then the ego mind has no chance. It is imperative then to focus away from the opponent, slightly to the side so that the mind is not captured by the ten thousand things and is operating within the domain of po.

All training in Taiji is with access to po as the highest consideration. The slowness of training, especially in the form, functions to create a state of boredom, which the self-aggrandizing ego cannot tolerate and will seek to escape allowing po to be predominant.

It is important to remember that fighting sequences when practiced solo should have this visualization of the opponent as a centerpiece of the practice. When practiced with a partner it should be done with the softness and serenity that is the Taiji form. To keep push hands from degrading into an aggressive version of hand-to-hand combat, the opponent should not be viewed directly. This is a practice for developing ting jing. Push hands has little if any actual street value. It is a mistake to think that push hands will carry over into the street. It is the value of ting jing that you learn through push hands that will serve you, and all efforts should be made to increase this. It is better to lose at push hands and gain in ting jing because that is where the real gain is to be found because then you are training po.

In fa jin, it is also necessary to train po. The fact that the candle has soothing effect on the practitioner and is itself a neutral object tends to increase the accessibility of po. All tendencies toward emotion such as shasi qi (killing air) should be avoided. The imaging used at the candle to delineate the opponent should be neutral and any attempt at effort or excessive force should be avoided.

This training is to build within you the confidence in the techniques of Taiji, and your access to po, but it is a great leap of faith to accept that these soft techniques can in fact defeat the hard aggressive moves of a superiorly strong individual. This is where the work of lazhu fangfa is important.

8-3 Using the Breath to Lead the Qi

Reverse Taoist breathing is used in lazhu fangfa to enhance the storage capabilities of energy on the inhale end of the cycle. This results in tensioning of the fascia of the abdominal area. The qi ball is formed by the downward thrust of the fascia, tendons, ligaments and muscles in the front section of the abdominal area. The inhale is accompanied by visualization techniques, which assist in leading the qi inward on the storage phase. This visualization consists of having the mental imagery of a contraction of tissues, muscle, tendon, ligament and fascia, which moves inward from the finger tips to the yongchuan of the rear foot. The sense that a pulse of energy created by this contraction is mentally moved from the fingers to the foot and is then followed by the void left by the relaxation of these contractions is extremely important. Wherever muscles are contracted, qi will fill that area. It naturally migrates to an area of muscular activity. It is as if the qi moved in to fill the void left behind by the contraction.

Visualizations, even when not accompanied by active muscular movement, involve minute contractions that accompany the imagery. With time and practice, these minute contractions can be enhanced and further increase the effect of the visualizations. This means that the technique of leading the qi with the breath can be practiced anywhere and at any time. It is not necessary to work at the candle for this to be an effective method and it is not actually necessary to perform the technique to train it.

8-4 Reverse Taoist Breathing

Reverse Taoist breathing functions as an additive pulse of energy, which combines, with the pulse already moving through the passages of the nine pearls, and with the proper timing, following the visualizations of the inward breath, it can enhance the existing pulse. Generally, the inhale will occur on the interception sequence and storage of energy, breathing will be coordinated with this interception, and the energy borrowed from it.

Reverse Taoist breathing is at its greatest efficiency when the epiglottis is closed and a vacuum created by the downward pull of the diaphragm is felt as a ball in the throat this is caused by the internal pressure within the mouth exerting a force against the epiglottis. This internal pressure is a result of this pressure differential This sensation of a ball in the throat is a general indication of the amount of effort or strength of the storage and also serves as a means of coordinating the contraction with the inhale, it also indicates that the contraction has occurred in the diaphragm, fascia, etc. In the early stages of this training, feedback is very important.

The actual function of Reverse Taoist breathing is in the storage and release of energy within the fascia, tendons and ligaments of the diaphragm, intercostal muscles and structures within the abdominal cavity. Reverse Taoist Breathing creates a tensioning of these systems in much the same way as muscle tone prepares the body for quick and powerful movements. This form of breathing is not stressed as much as it should be. It is essential for the performance of Hua Jing, the highest level of fa jin. The coordination of inhale and the contraction of the diaphragm with opening and closing (inhale should be on opening) results in a release that is explosive. This results from the compression of the time interval for the release. It is compressed by the fact that inhaling prevents the release of energy until an instant before the stoppage of the extremity in the performance of fa jin. The simplest way of generating this tension within the method of Reverse Taoist Breathing is by means of heng and haw. These are utterances that if done right can enhance efforts at hua jing. The vocalizations so common with Bruce Lee are nothing more than heng and haw. These sounds are a means of storing energy by virtue of Reverse Taoist Breathing. The strangeness of the sound Bruce Lee made was because it was developed on inhale, which gives you a distinctly different sound than on exhale.

8-5 Developing the Nine Pearls

Before performing lazhu fangfa, it is helpful to utilize the qi gong exercises that enhance feedback from the nine pearls. This assists the connection necessary for a continuous pathway for the intake and output of qi. The nine pearls are a very subtle sense of connection. It is not a rigid maintenance of the connection, as this will affect the flexibility of the extremity. Rigidity affects the mobility and the speed at which you can perform. There is a fine line between connection and a rigid member. You must find this by practice at the candle.

Prior to each attempt at lazhu fangfa, it is helpful to perform the Zhang Zhuang exercise standing like a post. The forward thrust of the thumbs in the two hand positions can facilitate this connection. This is the posture within the ma pu stance with hands in front, as if you were embracing a tree. It is over time that this connection of the nine pearls will become natural. Eventually, this connection will be the way you move through life, and you will be naturally very connected and very powerful. Whole body power will be at your finger tips at all times. It is possible to be connected and to be song.

If you experience joint pain, it is probably because you have not properly connected that joint, and an incomplete release at the candle will cause a rebound that will be expressed at the first incomplete connection. Use this pain to train in the proper connection, but also back off on the amount of power you are expressing at the candle until you have improved this connection.

8-6 Threading the Qi

The qi must be actively moved through the pathways of the body. Some passages are difficult to maneuver and require some unique methods to deliver it to the fingertips. After the second compression and bounce and in time with it, the yongchuan should be strummed. This is not a simple matter of pressing down on the yongchuan point. This must be a lifting of the leg by the downward pressure such that it presses the hip upward. It is as if you were to reach for some object on the upper shelves and had to stretch for it. This is accomplished without actually lifting the foot off the floor. The purpose of the strumming is the connection of the first three of the nine pearls. There is a second movement of the rear foot that is in conjunction with the strumming. This is a torque of the ankle with the yongchan as a pivotal point. This torque actually twists the hips in the direction that they have already been rotated by the first and second compressions. This is a further compression of the rotation and is timed with the bounce from the second compression.

The twisting of the hips and combined strumming thrusts the hips forward from the second bow to the arc of the third bow. The yongchuan of the third bow (forward foot) is pressed and the thread of qi is moved upward to the sacral pump. At the same time as the hips are thrust forward, the waist is turned in the direction of the candle; the hand maintains its centered position following along with the waist. It is when the hand is centered on the candle that the yongchuan of the forward foot is pressed and the hand is then thrust forward from the momentum of the forward thrust of the hips.

The sacral pump is activated to force the thread of qi through this difficult passage and into the spinal area. The pressure from the sacral pump and the qi belt must be combined to get the qi to move through this area. This means that as the sacral pump is pressed, there must be an upward thrust of the breath at the backside of the qi ball, which fans out through the qi belt to combine with the sacral pump and thus move the thread of qi through this area to the spine. The contraction of the qi belt begins with the upward thrust of the breath and moves from in front of the qi ball along the qi belt to the sacral pump where it is then compressed and moved upward to the spine.

The movement upward along the spine is facilitated by minute contractions of the musculature at the spine. All the muscle attachments at the spine are sequentially contracted to lead the qi upwards to the ming men. This is developed with feedback from the sensations of movement within the spinal area. It is a continuation of the thrust from the sacral pump and the upward thrust is maintained with the spinal contractions. The ming men or life's gate is activated when the thread of qi reaches there and contractions lead it into the shoulder area. Opening and closing move the thread across the shoulder area and the raised shoulders and hollowed chest move it into the arms. The energy stored with the rounded curves of the beautiful lady's hand, yu nu shou, thrust the energy forward by straightening this curve and the sudden stop at the candle combined with the strumming of the forward foot creates the release of qi at the fingertips.

8-7 Learning Whole Body Power with Lazhu Fangfa

Whole body power differs from an jing and fa jin in that whole body power is the same thing with out the release of qi at the extremities of the body into the opponent body. Whole body power is used to move the mass of the opponent in a specific direction to accomplish a technique. The waist is rotated and the qi is threaded through the body in the same manner as it is with the striking forces. Its use is in moving the opponent with in grasping situations, or with bodily contact, and the application of techniques with irresistible force, and the use of qi in a throwing or rooting application.

It is important to note that the techniques for the striking and the whole body applications are the same at the lazhu. It is only in the release of qi that they differ. This means that training for the striking applications is also training for whole body power. It is only a matter of applying the feed back learned from lazhu fangfa to the whole body power application.

8-8 Using the Lazhu to Train Qi Release

This practice utilizes two candles. It probably would be a good idea to use two candles through out the training. Quite often, the focus of your efforts will go beyond the first candle and then the one placed behind it will be extinguished. It may be appropriate to move the first candle a greater distance from the fingertips if it is not going out, and then you may hear a resounding pop because of the increase in power required to extinguish it. Another difficulty that can occur is the location or placement of your hand on release. If you release somewhat below the candle flame and at the candle itself instead of the flame, this can create difficulty in extinguishing the flame. At all times it is necessary to observe the direction of the force being applied. In order for the candle to be extinguished, the energy must be directed to the candle flame. This may seem obvious, but at the end of the strike, many students will flip the hand and the direction the force is moving is not in the direction of the candle flame.

The purpose of using the candle is to give the practitioner as much feedback as possible. It is therefore very important to use proper techniques so that this can be optimized. The release of qi at the candle without having it rebound back into your body is imperative. The rebound itself can cause damage at any of the nine pearls and probably as important: it can lead to a reduced power in the fa jin. This loss of power can be devastating in a martial application.

The release of qi in fa jin is one of stoppage of a forceful and physically developed energy pulse. This is accomplished by abruptly stopping the hand and allowing the pulse to continue. This is limited in scope, although it is effective, it does not maximize the power inherent in the internal process. To maximize the effects of qi, it is necessary to minimize the physical effort involved and use visualization to lead the qi from the fingertips to the yongchuan in the storage phase and reverse the direction and move the thread of qi upward to the fingertips on the emission phase. All movements that have been expressed before are now only visualized during the storage and emission phases, with one exception, the reverse Taoist breathing is emphasized and actively done to maximize the effects of the breath.

Begin by visualizing the energy moving in through the fingertips, down the arms to the ming men, to the hips, and through the heel to the yongchuan. This is done without actively trying to move each member: just placing the attention there is sufficient. Remember, that by placing your attention on a particular part of your body will result in minuscule movement and contractions of that area, which will mimic the actual performance as visualized. This maximizes the amount of effort relative to the strike that is contributed by the breathing cycle. Continual practice will create a sensation of a push of the energy through the body. This should be emphasized and enhanced.

Over time, this will increase the power of the strike and reduce the amount of physical effort required to produce it. This is important because the power produced places an enormous burden on the body. Tendinitis, cramps, and joint problems can occur when the body is over stressed.

8-9 Methodology of Different Strikes

There are several directional components to each individual strike. One component of hand movement is the application of a force in the opposite direction of the target on the storage phase of the sequence. This follows the rule that if you wish to move right you must first move left. If the interval between storage and the release of qi is short, then this will ensure that you are song. This component works because you allow the hand to continue on its storage path and rotate the waist in the direction of the forward foot before the backward moving hand is stopped. This causes the shoulder attachment and the waist rotation to be the driving force forward instead of the musculature.

There is another directional component that has as its reference point the application of a compressive force in toward the center of the body. This is the inward compression of the imaginary ball held between the hand and chest on the storage phase there is a third component, which is referenced by the character of the strike. If it is a vertical strike and does not strike directly down on top of the target, it is necessary to convert this vertical tangential force into a horizontal one in order to direct the force into the body. Even a horizontal circular force as in ward off needs a directional change in order to convert this circular energy with its angular momentum into a linear force to enter the target. In both instances, this is accomplished by the forward thrust of the hips at the third bow.

To understand each individual strike it is necessary to consider the direction of movement of the energy within the strike as it enters the body. The qi will follow the movement of the body, and it is therefore necessary to align the body movement with the target. The force generated is not the energy of a moving mass, but it is a sine wave similar to a cracked whip. If you strike some one with the middle of the whip with a downward thrust, all of the effect of the acceleration at the tip is lost.

8-10 Combining the Fighting Sequence and Lazhu fangfa

The strikes present within the particular fighting sequence you are using can be trained at the candle so that the proper steps, distancing and storage of energy can be practiced. The retreating sequences such as repulse the monkey should not be practiced before the candle since they are much more difficult to use in generating power for fa jin because the directional component is in the opposite direction and moves you away from the candle.

Fighting sequences, which are short forms designed for limited combat training can be practiced at the candle by taking out various portions of it in order to combine the stepping and the release of fa jin at the candle.

8-11 Ming Jing, An Jing and Hua Jing

There are three levels of force generated by fa jin. The lowest level of force generated and considered just a step above external force, is ming jing. This fa jin is accomplished by large circles, forceful storage of energy, and gross movement of qi. It is a learning stage and as such, it serves to assist in the transfer of external power to one of internal and soft power. It is a means of training the body in generation of high levels of energy with minimal muscular effort. It trains the mind in the acceptance of the possibility of soft force. The tendons, ligaments, sinews, fascia and all other parts of the body are strengthened by this utilization of gross movements with little muscular effort. The sequence of movements required to generate this explosive force of fa jin are also memorized.

An jing is the refinement of ming jing, which means visible force. An jing means hidden force. It is a more subtle version of the gross movements of ming jing. This is trained in two ways and then effort is made to combine the two separate methods. The first method is with gross movements such as in ming jing, but with gradual reduction in force applied so that eventually the large circular movements are reduced and effort at storage and emission at the candle is minimal. The second approach is to reduce the large movements gradually until the approach becomes imperceptible, but increasing the effort at storage and emission so that the candle can be extinguished. Eventually one should arrive at the place where it is possible to extinguish the candle with little motion and little effort at storage and emission.

There is not a clear distinction between these three levels of force. It is more of a continuum or gradation of one level into another. The final level, hua jing is called the perfect force. It is beyond the imperceptible motion of an jing, and is the elimination of motion in generating the force, and it is a result of yi yi yin qi. This translates as the mind leads the qi. It is the mental storage and movement of qi through the body and the mental expression of the energy at the fingertips. All movement is generated by visualization techniques and the minute muscular movements caused by the visualizations are imperceptible. At its highest level it is simply, the movements of qi by the po at the discretion of the yi mind.

9

Hand Striking Methods

9-1 The Circular Structure of Fa jin

There are certain axioms that are common to all varieties of empty hand striking methods within the internal styles. One of these fundamental truths is that all strikes are in the form of circles. This is true even for those that have the appearance of being straight or so brief that they apparently could only be straight. It is important to begin with large circles so that the circular concept is deeply embedded in the movement. It is important not to think of this as a linear striking method so that these circular aspects are not lost. Each particular hand strike has its own individual sequence of circular movements that develop the forces of fa jin. Within each of these circles are directional forces of either storage or energy emission. The gain from circular strikes is from the angular momentum increased by virtue of the distance off or the length of the radius, i.e. the farther the fist is from the body the greater the distance traveled on the outer circle. The distance traveled on the outer radius is greater for the same time interval. This translates as greater velocity. This can be visualized by using the imagery of a wagon wheel. The hub and the outer rim complete one rotation at the same time, yet the distance traveled on the outer rim is greater and therefore at a higher velocity.

These circular movements of the strike occur on a horizontal plane, vertical plane and even on a diagonal plane. There may be various combinations of the different planes such that a movement may be on a horizontal plane then a vertical plane and then a diagonal plane. It is also possible for the waist to be moving in one direction and the hand moving in another. These movements can be complicated and difficult to follow. Each movement does have a specific function that is important to developing the forces of fa jin. The arrow of direction of these circular movements will be described as if one was looking down on top of the individual from a point overhead. The arrow of direction will be either clockwise or counterclockwise from that vantage point.

Every circle has a center point and a radius that circumscribes the circle. The velocity of the hand can vary depending on the length of this radius as the waist is rotated. It is important to be cognizant of the distance off from the adept's body that the hand is at each juncture point. In describing these circular accelerations, it is necessary to use a standard method.

Each circle can be subdivided into an offensive arc, defensive arc or storage arc. An offensive arc is in the direction away from the body and directed at the center or about the center of the opponent for purposes of fa jin or an jing. Defensive arcs are directed generally toward an extremity or an off line portion of the torso for purposes of moving the extremity or body of the opponent to protect oneself. Offensive arcs are directed in toward the body of the protagonist and storage arcs are characterized by the arrow of direction of the energy moving in the direction of the body of the Taiji adept attempting the technique. This storage is for later or immediate release depending on the nature of the technique. The hand technique that is a good example of this is the straight chop. The hand actually follows a very shallow curve sideways toward the center plane of the body and then away when it is utilized for fa jin. This arc is in addition to the natural downward arcing movement of the striking hand, and is perpendicular to the normal striking arc. This is a compression of the force in an inward direction, which assists in the maintenance of the continuity of the force. This has the effect of increasing the available energy for fa jin by the use of angular momentum stored in these curvatures. All forces of whole body energy accumulate and are released with fang song gong to ensure an unobstructed pathway to the emission point.

At the same moment that the chopping strike is making these two arcs, one on the vertical plane and the other perpendicular, there is a forward-moving arc of the shoulder created by the rotation of the waist and the thrusting of the hips forward by the third bow. Each individual strike has its own individual eccentricity with respect to technique.

9-2 The Directionality of the Pulse of Energy

The combination of connecting the nine pearls and the inhale cycle of reverse Taoist breathing creates the sensation of an inward pulse of energy. This pulse is due to the sequential contractions of the tendons and smooth muscles at the tendon attachments of the nine pearls. The sequence of contraction at the nine pearls is from the designated hand through the wrist, up the arm, across the shoulder and down the spine and then to the yongchuan point. A rigid contraction of the musculature as in the "golden bell cover" is counter productive. It is a pulse of contractions that do no more than make the connection at each pearl a firm connection. A rigid contraction of the muscles will hinder movement and make the adept vulnerable to attack. Flexibility is paramount. This is a part of the storage phase of the fa jin cycle. It should be noted that this pulse is not actually the movement of qi, but is instead the contractions of muscles that lead the qi through the body.

Chu shou, bu chu zhou, admonishes you to move the hand out, not the elbow. This phrase common to Taiji expresses the need to follow the direction of the energy in the movement of a push outward from the body. In this instance, if your arm was pinned against your chest by the opponent, then you do not lead with your elbow in moving the arm. The elbow follows the lead of the hand. This can be practiced by having someone pin with two hands, your arm against the chest. If you lead with the elbow in pushing your arm away from the body, it becomes force against force. If you then spread your fingers and lead your movement and the movement of qi in the direction of your fingertips, it is no longer force against force. The amount of effort is reduced and the flow of qi is enhanced.

9-3 Cultivating the Minuscule Movements

Learning is intimately tied to muscle movement. The very first efforts of a newborn are in the area of gaining muscular control so that it can manipulate the environment. Our first efforts at reading are perusing the letters for recognition, tracing the letters, and memorizing these muscle movements. It is the initial muscle movements that are representations or symbols that are stored in memory. It is only later that the symbols are independent of the muscle movements. It would seem that they never are totally separated, but their role is minimized later on.

We begin our training in lazhu fangfa with gross circular movements and refine these until ultimately we have reduced the movements to their minimum. It is at this stage then that we must begin to refine those internal muscular movements we use in qi transport. This is done by relinquishing the effort to extinguish the candle for a period of time. It is is very difficult to reduce effort and intent when you have a goal of forcefully extinguishing the candle. It is by relinquishing this goal that we free ourselves from the control of the wisdom mind. You will still be able to cause the candle to flicker.

We can replace the attempts at extinguishing the candle with one of extending the time of the displacement of the candle flame. The longer the candle flutters in the onslaught of qi, then the more successful you are. This has the effect of taking the burden of extinguishing the candle and replacing it with one that is less demanding, yet it is in many ways more difficult. It means that you must produce more qi over a longer period of time. It removes that time compression needed for an explosive release of qi and additionally removes that ego-intent-demand for a forceful extinquishing of the flame.

9-4 Levels of Force in Striking

The initial attempts at fa jin will be mostly attempts at storage of a large amount of energy within the muscles. This is called local qi and it will be an assist until the actual movement of qi occurs with constant practice. Ming jing will have a large component of local qi in the early portions of training. As you move into an jing the level of local qi is reduced and the level of muscular tension with it. Within an jing the forces creating fa jin are internalized and although the movements are reduced and muscle tension is reduced, there is still an element of tension keeping you from being completely song. It is by relying on visualizations within hua jing that one can become song.

9-5 Visualizing the Minuscule

As we advance from learning muscle movements to the learning of symbolic muscle movements that accompanied the original learning and are associated with it, then visualizations will be remembered with it. We can take advantage of this by training large gross movements at first and then refining them and then eventually transferring this to a visualization technique, which is just as effective as the actual technique itself. What this means is that we will eventually with considerable effort; begin to transfer this memory of, and movement of the muscles, to one of a visualization of the movement. The visualization removes the ego mind from the equation and it is po moving the qi at the direction of the yi mind.

9-6 The Release of Qi

The release of qi at the candle is distinctly different from what actually occurs in a fa jin strike. This difference occurs because there is no object to stop the strike in lazhu fangfa. It is necessary then to deliberately stop the striking hand at the proper distance from the candle. This abrupt stop results in a rebound of the hand in ming jing and an jing. There is no rebound of the hand in hua jing, which is one of the ways in which you can characterize hua jing. Within hua jing there is a gentle stop of the hand because there is no need to remove forcibly the qi from the fingertips.

9-7 Force Differences between Fa jin and Hua Jing

There is within fa jin a large kinetic energy component accompanying a smaller qi component. Most of the energy derived from fa jin is of the kinetic variety. It is enhanced by the addition of qi, which results in the explosive power of fa jin. The accelerations derived by additive power of the various circular accelerations drastically enhance fa jin even before the enhancement by qi. The advantage of hua jing is not in the greater enhancement of energy, but by virtue of the fact that there is relatively little effort at generating it. This enhances one's endurance and serves to assist the concealment of intentions and actual delivery of hua jing. The concealment of your intentions and methods serves to destroy the opponent's strategy in that he has no way to discern your means of creating and delivering force. His confusion destroys his strategy and strengthens your ability by creating a superior tactical position. This is evident within your own practice when you as the one developing the energy, are surprised by its appearance.

9-8 Fatal Flute and Empty Hand

The highest level of development of lazhu fangfa is the ability to extend your qi to the tip of your weapon (see figure 9). In ancient China there was a saying within the community of martial artists, "if the flute is brought out, then someone is going to die." Those who used it did so with very subtle intent. It does not have the threatening significance of many weapons, and is easily concealed. It does not elicit the defensiveness in the opponent that many obvious weapons do.

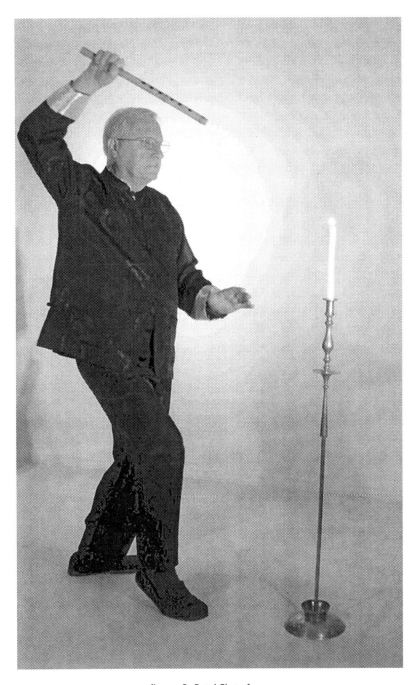

figure 9. Fatal Flute form

For purposes of learning to extend your qi to the tip of the weapon within the confines of lazhu fangfa, the fatal flute is ideal. It is a short weapon and results will be immediate. It is difficult to move the qi to the end of the straight Taiji sword because of its length. By initially starting out with a short weapon and then progressing to greater lengths, we can gain results in a very short period of time. The quicker you can extend the qi to your weapon tips, the greater the gain in your hand techniques. If you can extend the qi to the tip of a weapon, then the force and control of your hand techniques will be greatly magnified.

10

Striking from the Peng Position

10-1 Striking in Ward Off

The ward off position is the precursor for all hand strikes. It is the lesson learned from this position that is carried forward and is a determinant in the development of other strikes. It is then very important to develop, to the best of ones ability, the peng position strikes and energy dispersal. There are several factors involved in enhancing striking capabilities. These factors are; centering; being centered; chan sichou; nine pearls; the three bows; sacral pump; adhering the qi to the spine, and the hand circles. We are concerned here with the hand circles. The rest have already been discussed in earlier chapters.

In Taiji, circular movement is of critical importance in generating the force of fa jin. Straight line movements do not create the angular momentum and the accelerations caused by circular movement. These all have been discussed, but what has not been discussed is this minuscule acceleration that occurs at the movement of the hand itself. Considering that you have initiated fa jin from the peng position with circular movements and you have done everything right as presented so far, then if you assume this should be the complete technical aspects of the form of fa jin for this posture, you would be wrong. For every type of strike there is a distinctive circular hand function that should occur at the moment of the strike that is specific to that particular hand strike. With the peng posture, it is the beautiful lady's hand that is in operation as a circular hand function. It has been mentioned earlier, but the mechanics of the circular functions were not described because the subject has already become very complicated. Fa jin is not a simple straight forward punch as in most martial arts. It is of a complexity unparalleled in the martial world. To simplify and categorize the striking differences, the arc formed by the hand is described in detail and the energy storage potentials are treated in detail for each striking method.

The arrow of direction of fa jin is critical in determining the other arrows of energy direction. For instance, in peng the arrow of direction of fa jin is on the horizontal plane and moves forward from the centerline of the practitioner into the centerline of the opponent. All of the rotational energies of chan sichou and the turning of the waist deliver the qi to the hand at the centerline and these would be dissipated within the surface of body if it were not for the forward thrust of the hips, which translate this circular energy into a forward thrust and into the body of the opponent. It is important that you realize that the direction of motion of the energy is tangential to the arc formed by the hand and until this change of direction by the thrusting of the hips toward the candle, the energy is moving away from the candle in the direction of rotation. Much of the energy lost in fa jin attempts is due to the misapplication of the arc of the striking hand with reference to direction. The energy must be applied in the direction of the target, from centerline of the practitioner to the centerline of the opponent. We know that the strike is always in that direction, but without comparing the energy arriving to the direction it is supposed to go, we do not know if we have completed the necessary cycle. This transfer of rotational energy into linear energy toward the candle is essential to maintain the proper power.

It is the pulse of energy moving from the yongchuan out the arm that straightens the curvature of the beautiful lady's hand somewhat changing the diameter of the circle of the striking hand so that it is on the outer circle, thus increasing the velocity of the hand. It is important within the dynamics of this hand curvature that the movements from the inner circle are not the result of the muscles of the upper body, but due to the energy of the pulse and the turning of the waist. This is consistent with being song to allow the free flow of energy.

The particular hand arc that we are concerned with at this time is the arc of compression. Each of the hand strikes has a compression cycle, which is in essence a function of the concept, "if you want to move right, then you must first move left." Holding the ball and compressing the ball inward in the peng position is in a sense creating an opposing arc for the striking hand, which is a storage method. The release of this compression is another additive force that combines with the pulse of fa jin. This can best be described by visualizing holding a large beach ball with one arm and compressing it against your chest. When you release this pressure, the hand and the ball tend to bounce away from you.

The end result of all this is that there are three arcs of motion that the hand describes in striking a target. The first arc is a precursor to the strike and is an arc of compression and storage of energy in the opposite direction to which the hand will finally move. It is a horizontal arc and the center of the circle forming the arc is the tantien. The second arc is made in conjunction with the forward strike of the hand and is a compression of the hand inward toward the body with the center of the circle at the center of the opponent's body. The third arc is the release of energy and the relaxation of all tensions resulting in the vertical arc of the hand caused by the forward thrust of the hips and the combined direction from the other arcs. The center of this circle is the ming men point

10-2 The Circles of Peng

The movement of energy through the body must be in the form of whole body power. This is accomplished by the circular motion of the extremities all moving in conjunction with the body as a unit, and when you use the hand as a reference point itself in describing these circles, then it begins to make sense. The motions of the hand are as if it is rigidly connected to the center of the body by an iron bar, and the body moves with the hand on the centerline of the body where maximum power can be generated. It also moves in coordination with the movements of the body and does not move independently of it. The muscles of the upper torso are not used to move the hands. It is from the movements generated by the waist, hips and chan sichou that the hand moves. The precise coordination of bodily movements with the circles created by the hand movements is a result of the conscious engagement of the nine pearls. One of the circles in the peng position is the beautiful lady's hand. It is circular in form in its structure. It is caused by the natural arc formed by the graceful curvature, and as such stores the angular moment, which is released by the slight straightening of the arm and forearm. The hand should not go beyond a mere straightening of the wrist, if it does a large amount of stress will be placed on the wrist and damage can result from the hinge action of the wrist.

Rotating the waist with the hand located in a position in close to the body results in an additional acceleration when the hand moves out into a circle with a longer radius. The acceleration is caused by the increased distance along this outer circle covered in the same rotation interval of the waist on the inner circle. This has increased proportionally the distance traveled on the outer circle. This is mathematically proportional to the increase in the length of the radius. The net effect is to double the velocity of the hand on the outer circle. Added to this is the acceleration caused by the forward thrust of the hips. These are accumulative forces similar to being in a car and throwing a ball forward. The final circle is the rotation of the hand and the release by the beautiful lady's hand.

10-3 The Timing of Peng

The precise timing of events within the strike from the peng position is critical to the strength of the pulse delivered. The events that are critical to timing are as follows in order of occurrence: inhale; first four of the nine pearls; beautiful lady's hand; closing; rotate the waist toward the rear foot and hollow the chest as you contract the diaphragm in reverse Taoist breathing; maintain the hand on the centerline; compression of the leg muscles by torsion; balance is maintained over yongchuan by pressing downward and lifting the hip with this motion; compression of the sacral pump; contraction of qi belt and intercostal muscles; rotation of the waist away from the rear foot; breathe out; maintain hand on the centerline; rotation stops when the hand is aligned with opponents center line; thrust forward with hips; bounce weight off front foot; breathe out; stop hand. There is a thread of continuity that must be maintained so that the pulse is amplified by constructive interference and is not interrupted or decreased by destructive interference. This is why it is critical to be song. The energy must be free flowing in the direction of the hand and not be dispersed within the body of the adept.

10-4 The Storage Sequence

The storage sequence can begin with the interception of the opponents hand or not, depending on the circumstances. If interception is the case, then the storage cycle begins with borrowing energy from the opponent. If it does not begin with interception, then it begins with the visualization of energy moving inward, from the hand to be used in striking through the nine pearls. This must occur in conjunction with inhale cycle of reverse Taoist breathing. Yu nu shou or beautiful lady's hand must also be evident. This means that energy must be stored in the curvature of the arm, forearm and hand. Straightening this curvature of the arm will release the stored energy, in much the same manner as a bowed branch snaps forcefully back when released.

The rotation of the waist is passive in nature, but the storage of energy derived from it in the form of chan sichou is not passive. It is passive in its formation, but it must be actively generated by the contraction of the leg muscles in this area in order to compress and drive the energy in the opposite direction (forward). In the same manner as energy is stored in chan sichou, the rippling of the spine in the storage phase is passive, but there must be active contractions that straighten the spine as in the "beautiful ladies hand" which discharges the energy stored in the structures.

10-5 Chan Sichou

Chan sichou occurs in the storage phase of fa jin. It results from the twisting of muscular tissue as the waist is rotated, either by the force of interception or by the active rotation for storage purposes. This occurs first in the waist as it is rotated and then the muscles of the back and stomach are twisted and compressed by the rotation. The muscles of the leg are twisted by the rotation with the rear foot planted, restricting the rotation of the leg and waist. You can increase this effect by contracting the muscles of the leg and waist. This contraction magnifies the storage effect of chan sichou.

10-6 The Energy Pulse

The literature of the Taiji classics reveals that when you deliver force into the opponent you must push the qi to the end of all the hairs in the body. In order to generate real power from the fa jin strike, it is necessary to understand the principles behind this statement. This push, as the ancients called it, is a coordinated compression of the muscles of the body, which moves a sine wave of energy through the body to the hands, foot or other extremity. A good analogy would be to compare it to squeezing a tube of toothpaste. You start at the bottom and move the paste toward the opening and without allowing the paste to get behind the point at which you are currently squeezing. This ensures that there is no paste, i.e., energy loss. This requires that you to deliver the qi forward without any loss at each of the various nine pearl locations of difficult transition.

The energy that we have deliberately stored in the curvatures of the body will be lost through out the body unless we control the manner in which this dispersal occurs. We do not want a uniform distribution of the energy of fa jin throughout the body. We have to direct the energy pulse along predetermined channels to a specific end point of our choosing. This is accomplished by managing this pulse of energy with minuscule contractions that direct the final dispersal. The qi is gradually kneaded upward toward the extremity while being contained so that it does not move in an undesirable direction. The squeezing of the pulse is readily discernible, but this control of the energy pulse is not.

One of these methods of controlling the dispersal of energy of fa jin is the cranial pump. The cranial pump consists of the contraction of the muscles in the temporal region. If you place your fingertips on the temporal area and clench your teeth, you can feel the contraction of this muscle group. One of the postural items that all forms of Taiji utilize is that of placing the tongue on the gum line just behind the front teeth. The purpose behind this technique is that of energy distribution. If the energy pulse moves up to the head area it will spit into two directions. One pathway is up the back of the head to the top of the crown, and the other is up the front through the tongue and across the face to the crown. These two forces meet head on and effectively neutralize each other. This also prevents any additional energy of the pulse from moving in this direction. The pulse is then forced to move from the ming men into the shoulder and out to the extremity.

We are starting with the tongue on the gums first which is the reverse direction for the pulse because it is important to have all of these connections in place prior to strumming the yongchuan. In reverse order of the actual pulse, the next consideration is the intercostal connection at the spinal column.

Visualizing the energy moving inward from the hand and forming the nine pearls in the storage phase prepares the pathway for the energy pulse as it returns through the body in a combined form. This combination of the energy pulse begins with the strumming of the yongchuan point. The lifting action of the yongchuan combined with the torque of the ankle drives the pulse upward to the hip. The torque of the ankle serves to make the leg one rigid piece that allows the energy to travel this pathway. It is difficult to move the energy pulse across the pelvic girdle. It is therefore necessary to utilize the sacral pump to accomplish this. Contraction of the muscles around the sacrum will result in an almost imperceptible lifting of the sacrum. This is enough to transfer the pulse to the spine.

In conjunction with the transfer to the spine, there is a forward thrust of the hips moving the geometric center of mass closer to the yongchuan point on the forward foot. This allows a minor gravity drop with the shift forward and a reversal of the direction of the pulse resulting from the gravity drop, caused by the downward pressure onto the forward yongchuan point. This is not the same pulse as generated by the rear yongchuan, but is instead combined with it at the spine and constructive interference results in a greatly magnified pulse. It requires practice to combine these two pulses. They can be combined because the beginning pulse is delayed by the difficult passage through the hip area.

The pulse must be actively pushed with the musculature in the area it is moving. This is very much like squeezing a tube of toothpaste. It is even more important to squeeze it out of the forearm for complete release into the body of the opponent. There are five different but equally important sources of power: there are the accelerations from the circles of Taiji; secondly, there is the enhancement of the forces by the addition of qi; thirdly, there is whole body power, which accumulates energy by moving the body as a unit rather than individual parts moving separately. There is also the active push, which moves the qi through the body, and finally there is the timing of each individual event, which results in the accumulation of constructive interference and magnifies the force of all the separate energies. These simple procedures will do more for increasing the power of your strike than any other single thing. These are subtle, yet very dramatic means of increasing the force of fa jin.

10-7 Complete Sequence

Standing before the candle or lazhu with your hand before you, palm faces inward, and in the Taiji ready stance, visualize the opponent chambering his arm and striking forward toward you. This is the triggering event you have practiced with the soft ball and by visualization practice. It will cause you to enter into the warrior mind or po. This is essential since you will not always be aware that some one is attacking you and it is necessary to react immediately and without any decision making process.

The initial reaction is always defensive. It is necessary because your storage of energy comes from the defensive movements you make. It is possible to store qi and use it, but at this stage, it is the storage for fa jin that is critical. Your interception will be a circular movement upward and forward in a counterclockwise circular manner with your left intercepting hand with which you connect with the incoming fist at the inside of the wrist area. This contact should be at the top of the arc that your hand makes and the hand should be moving in the same direction as the incoming fist when this contact is made. The Taiji ready stance with the front toe raised will force you to have your weight balanced over your rear foot. It is very important that you train yourself to start from this position. Later when your technique is perfected, you can stand in a normal stance with your hands at your side. For this technique at this time, it will be necessary to move forward into the mountain climbing stance as you intercept. This will allow you to close the distance and it will prevent you from over extending beyond your circle of power. The distance away from your body for this circle of power can be determined by placing a stick along the shin of the rear foot. The interception point of your hand in the peng position and this stick is the distance off the circle of power.

As the hand is drawn in toward you, rotate the waist so the incoming opponents hand moves around you as you maintain the hand on the horizontal centerline. The rotation of the waist will create the storage of energy in the form of chan sichou in the waist and legs. You should be inhaling with reverse Taoist breathing. The strumming of the Yongchuan and the torque of the rear foot should activate the second bow, and compress the first three of the nine pearls already connected by sensing them on the interception. This compression of the twisted musculature and the three of the nine pearls sends a pulse of energy much like squeezing a tube of toothpaste. This should arrive at the sacrum and the activation of the sacral pump moves this up into the vertebral column.

Sequential contraction of the intercostal connections at the spine will send the pulse up to the ming men point and across the shoulder into the arm. The arm should have the contour adequately described as the beautiful lady's hand or yu nu shou. In conjunction with this, there is a forward movement into the mountain climbing stance. This is the third bow and it translates the movement from a circular one into a linear one moving in the direction of the candle.

The release is a circular motion of the beautiful lady's hand counter-clockwise and the straightening of the curvature of the beautiful lady's hand.

10-8 Analysis of Energy

The energy derived from this form of fa jin is a combination of angular momentum at different distances from the center and the constructive interference gained from combining three wave fronts with the first bow. One from the first bow and one from the second bow, and the third one from the pulse created by the exhale from reverse Taoist breathing. The final acceleration occurs when the beautiful lady's hand is released at the candle.

These accelerations result in an acceleration of this pulse, much as the sine wave accelerates down the length of a whip, and when it reaches the stiff end, the inflexible tip decreases the amplitude of the wave, while the frequency increases. This results in an acceleration of the tips of the fingers that exceed the speed of sound. It is this shock wave that results in a small sonic boom at the candle and extinguishes the flame. This sonic boom is evident in the pop of the candle flame as it is extinguished.

In addition to the energy of acceleration, there are minute muscular contractions that move the pulse up through the body. This produces a wave front that moves through the body. Qi will automatically gravitate to areas of muscular activity. It is similar to the metaphor of the stick drawing a line in the dirt and being filled by the water from the puddle. The mind cannot direct the qi, but it is possible to control the muscular contractions with the mind. This is an indirect way to control the flow of qi. One of the important things to do in practice is to learn to develop this sequential movement of the wave front by muscular contractions. It is through the musculature that this pulse moves. It is not across or through the bones that this wave pulse moves, but is instead through the muscles and across the tendons and ligaments at the joints. The nine pearls are created by the tensioning of these muscles at the end of the tendons and ligaments. It is by fixing the joints with these contractions that a pathway across them is created. This is not a rigid fixation of the joints, but is merely consists of holding in the joint in place with enough tension that a pathway is created across the tensed tendons and ligaments. It is the ability of the structures to flex under tension that creates this sine wave of force moving through the body. This is the same principle that occurs when we snap a clothesline and send a sine wave down its length. It is, however, closer to a violin string that is strummed and you send out these vibrations, except that it is one pulse sent to the unattached end at the extremity. The hand then serves as a transducer, which carries this pulse from the medium of muscle, tissue and bone into the air in the form of a sonic sound wave. A transducer is a device that transports an energy wave from one medium to another. Sonar for instance mechanically produces a sonic wave of a given frequency that is transferred across a plastic barrier into the water.

The explosive pop that we hear at the candle is this sonic boom created by the acceleration of the fingertips past the speed of sound. On the ground, we are at a distance from the airplane causing a sonic boom and there is a delay, but at the candle, the sound is immediate. It is difficult to determine whether the sound is from the fingertips as in the crack of the whip, or from the expulsion of the pool of wax at the base of the wick. There are many things that go into the accelerations. We know that humans can throw a baseball at one hundred miles an hour, and we know that moving the fist out onto the outer circle can double the velocity, and that the forward thrust is additive. These additions are then accumulated at the arm and the beautiful lady's hand, which like a whip creates a sine wave whose amplitude is compressed as it moves down its length. There is an inverse relationship between the amplitude and the velocity or frequency of the wave. As the amplitude decreases the velocity increases, and this creates the high velocity that leads to the sonic boom. Another analogy is the inbound wave at a shoreline with the low shallow wave amplitude and wide breadth of the wave building in height as it moves into the shallows. This is caused by the shores resistance to forward movement of the wave front. This tends to build the amplitude or the height of the wave to considerable magnitude and sends it crashing onto the beach with overwhelming force. This also represents that inverse relationship between velocity of the wave and amplitude.

In addition to these mechanically derived forces, there is the force of qi, which can be accelerated through the body. This wave of qi follows the induced sine wave and ads its energy to it. This energy is in the form of psychokinetic energy and is dismissed by much of the scientific community, but research by the Rhine Studies at Duke University indicates otherwise. The research itself cannot be contested on the basis of its technical and mathematical merit. In truth, those in the scientific community dealing with the philosophy of science state that if you invalidate the studies based on the statistical analysis, then the whole foundations of quantum mechanics must also be thrown out.

The final energy added to the systematic accelerations of this punch can be in the form of zhen jing or whole body power. This is not an acceleration of the forces of energy inherent in fa jin but is a result of moving the body in a coordinated manner so that the muscular forces developed can be delivered from the yongchuan to the tip of the fingers. This does not move at the speed of the pulse, but can be delivered after as a one two punch, only from the same hand. It occurs with the counter rotation of the hips and in conjunction with the foreword thrust of the hips. It is not a pulse of energy, but is, instead, a sustained movement of energy that will carry the individual with it. Whole body power is the moving of the body in a uniform and integrated way to deliver the force of body movement not an accelerated pulse to the opponent. The delivery hand is kept on the centerline at the most efficient place or position of power.

The result is that not only is a high velocity pulse delivered to the opponent, but also a coordinated moving mass is delivered right behind it. The strike has penetrating power and zhen jing has the ability to break the opponents root. Coordination of fa jin and whole body power yields an explosive force that overwhelms the opponent and drives him back with devastating force, and breaks his root, while at the same time it delivers penetrating power.

There are augmentations of this energy created by the coordination of breathing with the fa jin and zhen jing applications. Access to po can be developed by using the breath to coordinate fa jin and zhen jing. Availability of qi is directly related to access to po. It is po that controls the distribution of qi; Taiji is essentially a moving meditation. The augmentation of fa jin by the breath is a function of both the coordination of the various aspects of fa jin with the breath and the insertion of qi into the equation by the immediate access to po with its control of qi.

10-9 Sequential Breakdown

In step one of the strike from peng position, assume the mountain climbing stance with your right hand in the peng position and the hand approximately six inches from the candle. Visualize the opponent chambering his right arm in preparation for throwing a punch. This is the first access to po and should be trained by interception with the softball intercept at the top of the circle. Extend your left hand in an upward circular motion to intercept the incoming fist, at the inside of the wrist, and at the top of the arc with your hand moving back toward you at the time of intercept so that the hand is moving in the same direction as the opponents hand.

In step two, the breath should be drawn in with a thin cool stream of air, and the movement of the hand and the turning of the waist should be coordinated so that the hand remains on the adept's centerline. The breath is the second means of access to po for training purposes. The intercept was a trigger mechanism, which should cause the Taiji adept to move immediately from the state of hun or the ten thousand things to the state of po. By coordinating the breath and stilling the mind during training, we further reinforce this access to po. The Coordination of the breath with stilling of the mind is like marking the date on the wall with a hash mark is a good reminder to do this. It is a means of noting the passage of events.

Step three follows the breath by rotating the waist in coordination with the "reverse Taoist breathing." This breathing style compresses the abdominal area causing pneumatic and hydraulic compression within the body."Rolling the ball" occurs when the waist nears the end of its rotation toward the rear foot. This technique is a downward rotation on the outer portion of the abdomen, which will be followed by an upward rotation of the inner portion in the next step. This creates a directional flow to the pulse created by the combination of "rolling the ball" and "reverse Taoist breathing." The turning of the waist results in chan sichou, which is the storage of energy by the torsion and compression of muscles. This is similar to the twisting of a hemp rope, which creates a rigid piece.

Step four consists of strumming the yongchuan point on the ball of the rear foot. This strumming is an upward lift, which is much the same as if you were reaching for something on a high shelf. This is accompanied by an inward torque of the ankle that combines with the sequential contraction of the muscles of the calf and thigh to drive the pulse up to the hip area. Exhale should not begin until the waist is completely counter rotated and the hips are square with the candle. The pulse can be felt at the hip joint and passage to the spine is assisted by activating the sacral pump. Contractions of the sacral pump move the pulse to the spine in the sacral region up to the dorsi and latisimus dorsi muscle group, which contracts in sequence to move the pulse upward to the trapezius muscle group. The intercostal muscle groups also come into play to bridge the soft tissues of the waist area.

Step five is the movement of the pulse up the spine with sequential contractions of the dorsi, latisimus dorsi, trapezius muscles that move the pulse from the ming men to shoulder area.

The complete release of all fa jin derived energies at the candle is by a clockwise rotation of the arm as depicted by beautiful lady's hand. This release occurs on a forward thrust at the point the hand begins the upward stroke of the circular hand movement in the third bow so that fa jin occurs at that instant when the hand has begun its up ward movement. This causes a lifting moment and is instrumental in breaking the individuals root. Added to this as a coordinated assist, is the reverse Taoist breathing that characterizes the strike of fa jin. By compressing the abdomen on inhale, we are creating pneumatic and hydraulic pressures within the body. The release of these forces adds to the existing pulse and helps accelerate it.

10-10 Yin and Yang in Peng Strikes

In striking, the back of the hand is generally considered yang and palm of the hand is considered yin. This is not always the case. In palm strikes, the palm would be considered the action side or yang. In the storage phase of the strike cycle, the palm side also becomes the active side with respect to action and energy. This role is again reversed when the emission phase begins with the song release of energy.

10-11 Stringing the Bow and Drawing the Arrow

Often just stating the something in a different manner adds insight into a meaning or technique. The concept of stringing the bow is a means of looking at the storage of energy in the peng position that has some visualization benefit. If we are standing before the candle with an unstrung bow, then nothing will happen. If we think in terms of opening and closing as the means of stringing the bow, then it is easier to visualize what is happening. It takes considerable practice before the candle before you develop the muscular control necessary to make this complicated and some what subtle connection necessary to emit the full force of fa jin. Opening and closing is evident in the qi gong exercise Zhang Zhuang. When we are in the position of standing like a tree, this is a closing position. Our shoulders are raised, the arms are rounded and we are in the mountain climbing stance. As we move back and position our weight over our back foot, we move into an opening position by drawing back our arms and removing the hollow in our chest. In conjunction with this, we are rotating our waist toward the rear foot. A slight upward pressure on the yongchuan at the same time as we accomplish the opening exercise will string the bow. This will give the sensation of the two arms being strung together like a bow. With practice the subtle understanding of these individual elements will give considerable power to the total effort of fa jin.

Rotating the waist with a strung bow delivers the arrow or pulse of energy to the forward thrusting hips or the third bow, which will in turn accelerate it at the beautiful lady's hand.

10-12 Peng Jing in the Release from Hand Grips

Standard techniques such as used in chin na utilize the twisting and compression of joints and pinching nerves to gain a release or manipulate a grip of the opponent. Using fa jin entails manipulating the grip in such a manner that the explosive force of fa jin can be utilized or the softer contact force of an jing and can be employed for a release from a handgrip, to illustrate this, utilize a cross handgrip from the opponent that is for instance right-hand to right-hand. It is important to offer your hand in such a manner that the palm is facing down. This assures that you have maximum rotation capability. With the opponent gripping your right wrist, rotate your right hand horizontally (the axis of rotation is vertical through your hand) in the direction of the thumb for one half circle using your waist to generate the power for movement and the storage of energy for release in fa jin. Think of your palm resting on the top of a staff with the other end of the staff resting on the ground and then rotate your hand without the staff leaving the vertical position. This will rotate the opponent's wrist and arm. The addition of a slight counterclockwise rotation of the waist will result in unbalancing the opponent without uprooting him. The effect of this movement is twofold. First, the opponent's arm will be locked and it is possible to utilize it as one piece without it collapsing. You must then counter rotate his arm to the opponents left, while maintaining the lock. You will have the opponent in an arm bar which will allow you to deliver fa jin up his arm to his shoulder. Secondly, the back of the hand will be placed against the carpal tunnel ligaments of the wrist. The force of fa jin can then be released against this area and cause the release of the grip by the forward movement of the hand toward the opponent and the explosive force of fa jin. This force will not stop with the effects on the wrist but should continue up the stiff arm and be delivered to the shoulder of the opponent, moving him backward.

The direction of the force emitted should be toward the center of the opponent. If it is directed off the center then the arm could collapse and avoid the force. By committing the force to the center of the opponent, the opponent will be moved as if the force where directly applied to his center.

There are many different ways that these principles can be applied. It is only limited by your imagination. You should also train in a continuous flow from one technique to another, so that you are not trapped by a failed technique. It is also important not to apply a technique, but instead to utilize what is given by the opponent in the most efficient manner possible.

The energy pulse of fa jin has a disorienting effect on the opponent because it is unexpected and does not fit within the normal experience of an opponent. The individual has no idea what has happened or how it can be countered. This is a very disarming event and can be used psychologically to defuse a confrontation.

10-13 The Release

The release of energy at the candle is tricky because the momentum of the hand must be stopped abruptly without stopping the movement of the pulse to the fingertips. This pulse will rebound if it is not properly released. The pulse must be compressed into the fingertips at the point in which it is stopped. This is comparable to the crack of the whip, which is caused by the abrupt stopping of the forward moving hand, while at the same time the accelerating sine wave as the whip approaches the rigid tip. In order to be song and relaxed at the point of discharge of the pulse, it is necessary to learn to stop the forward movement of the hand without the rigid contraction of the arm and forearm. Any attempt at whipping the hand to discharge the energy is counter productive. This will defeat your efforts at being song, and interfere with the natural flow of energy, and can result in damage to the carpal tunnel area of the wrist. With practice, it becomes evident that the energy pulse will continue to flow outward naturally without expressly discharging it. Taiji is not a soft version of the external martial arts and should not be treated as such. In order to get beyond the range of twelve inches in extinguishing the candle, it is necessary to develop the release of qi while maintaining the state of song.

10-14 Combining Visualizations

An important part of each striking technique is the need to incorporate all the aspects and various visualizations with those other visualizations such as those in the form, the fighting sequence, the interception practice, and the practice at the candle. By combining them and making each one a factor in training, we make our practice effective in the real world. It is necessary, however, to merge these separate visualizations of the opponent and make sure that they are tied to each other and form a continuous whole. This is done by making certain that the visualizations impinge on po and not just the yi or wisdom mind. Yi yi yin qi means that the wisdom mind leads the qi, but it is only through its interaction with po that this occurs.

Training must be specific to po. This can be done for instance in interception and the fighting sequence by centering our attention away from the center of activity and making our peripheral vision central to our perception. The peripheral vision is the domain of po, while the fovea or focused center of vision is the domain of the yi mind.

Repetitive and ritualistic type training tends to promote access to po because the yi mind will escape the boredom at every opportunity.

The startle reflex and use of xiao qi or kia of the Japanese tends automatically to move the individual into a trance like state, which is in reality po. It is trance like by virtue of the fact that it is untrained and unresponsive, because po does not perceive the future or past; therefore it cannot interpret the nature of the threat. It operates on the basis of manipulating incoming and outgoing energies. It operates on the basis of the autonomic hard-wire preprogramming or intensive training of an internal art system like Taiji. Xiao qi is effective only on an untrained po.

Change is a window on po. Constant change and the learning process are effective means of access to po, because the yi mind abhors change. It does so because change is an unknown, and difficult for the yi mind to control. To maintain preeminence the yi mind prefers the known because the known is familiar and this eliminates fear, chaos, and the possibility that it would lose preeminence.

Po and the yi mind must be held close together. It is the yi mind that understands the world of the ten thousand things and therefore understands what is happening, but it is po that has the speed and precision necessary for effective application of techniques. It is also po that has access to qi. This is a formidable combination in the martial arena.

Serenity keeps po near while complexity (the phenomenal world) keeps yi near. It is by working from one to the other that we keep them in close contact. We are constantly testing to see that they are not far from each other.

It is at the candle that all these visualizations converge. The interception sequence with its visualization is practiced and all the visualizations of the form and fighting sequences are combined into one image of the opponent at the candle which culminates in the release of explosive force in the form of fa jin.

11

Alternate Striking Methods

11-1 Elements of the Chopping Strike

The openhanded chopping strike is the next point of discussion because it is very easy to see the various arcs formed by the hand in motion (see figure 10).

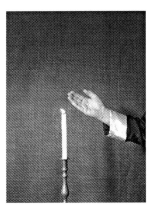

figure 10. Open hand chop

As with most Taiji, it begins with a defensive move, intercepting with the left hand, generally it is an interception triggered by the motions of the opponent. With proper training, this should cause the Taiji adept to enter into that realm of thought the Chinese call po. The chopping strike can be delivered by either peng or old ox power. When peng is the form of storage with a left hand intercept and a right hand strike and release there is a counter-clockwise (storage) and then a clockwise rotation (emission). When old ox power is used there is a counterclockwise (storage), and then a clockwise (also storage), and finally an additional clockwise rotation (emission). There is a second method of storage for old ox power fa jin which is more direct. This occurs when there is no interception with the left

149

hand. The rotation is then clockwise for the storage phase and then counterclockwise for the emission phase. The interception phase serves as a means of storage and interception at the same time. This yields reciprocity between the emissions of one hand and the storage of the opposing hand, such that yin and yang are continuous in the development of internal qi. Opening yields an opposing closing etc.

For purposes of simplification, the emission phase of the complete cycle will be stressed and only the arcs described by the hands will be considered. It should be understood that all of the other energy accumulations also apply when actually using fa jin.

The simplified storage phase will be used to describe the first arc. It is a storage phase in which the hand is raised on vertical line that is centered between the opponents centerline and the adepts. This places the hand on the most powerful position as determined earlier with the stick on the shin. As the hand is raised, there must be a resistance applied in the opposite direction to which the hand is raised. A practice for this is to place the other hand on the wrist and resist the raising of the striking hand until the idea is reinforced and occurs naturally.

The second arc is different from the emission phase of peng. In addition to being vertical rather than horizontal, it is not pulled by the shoulder and therefore requires additional effort to maintain continuity of the final three pearls. Instead of being pulled by the shoulder as it is driven by the waist movement, it is pushed by the forward movement of the shoulder. The change in elevation of the hand is therefore caused by a deliberate lowering of the hand. The final three pearls are maintained by compressing the vertical downward stroke in toward the center such that a shallow arc is described curving inward to the body. This structurally creates the one piece needed for continuity in the flow of qi.

The two arcs have the tantian as their center point. If you consider san guanxi and the positioning of hand, foot, elbow and knee, you will understand that this is an aid in locating the hand on the position of power. The inward compressing arc has its center point located somewhere in space considerable distance away at ninety degrees on a horizontal plane with the tantian.

To clarify this, you must understand that this strike is composed of two mutually operating arcs. One of these arcs is an arc formed by the vertical downward stroke of the hand with the shoulder as its source. The other arc is a shallow movement of the hand in an arc that is a sideward movement in an arc that stores energy in the form of closing and releases it upon striking. The purpose of this second arc is the inward pressure it causes storing energy in the opposite direction of the strike.

The result is a downward thrust composed of a series of small arcs. The first arc is the movement from the inner circle to the outer circle at the waist, magnifying the acceleration caused by the turning of the waist and moving the hand some distance from the center. Increasing the distance from the center increases the acceleration. This is a result of the increased distance traveled on the outer arc in the same period of time. The second acceleration in principle is the same as holding the ball with the hands. It is an inward compression and storage due to the techniques of closing. The third is a change of direction. It is a forward thrust, which changes the sideways force and vertical components into a thrust in the direction of the centerline of the opponent. This is accomplished by whole body power and the movement of the third bow.

The arrow of direction of the chopping strike using the tile hand is outward from the center, and in this case, the attachment point is the shoulder. It is the forward thrust of the hips in transferring the weight from the rear foot to the forward foot that moves the strike into the opponent, transferring the downward thrust into a forward movement into the opponent. This is a difficult maneuver since most people lose the concept of song and whole body power and tend to move the arm separately using muscles instead of the angular momentum derived from the waist and thrust of the hips.

The circles of acceleration in this strike are very different from the strike using the peng stance. The rotation of the waist in the storage phase is in conjunction with the raising of the hand and the storage of energy in the peng position, one of closing: while within the chopping strike, it is one of opening. This is an important distinction, since the arrow of direction of the energy in the storage phase is in the opposite direction. These are two distinct methods of storage, which will be discussed later. Because the storage phase is from opening, it naturally follows that the acceleration of the hand is initially from moving the waist toward the forward foot and the acceleration of the hand downward by closing and the addition of the forward thrust of the hips.

The forward thrust of the hips in the peng position causes the hand to sweep in a shallow curve upward toward the candle. The chopping strike is accelerated by the force of gravity, which will not give you nearly as much acceleration. To this downward pull of gravity is added a counter rotation to the rotation of the waist on its completion. The waist is rotated with the hand moving past the centerline with the candle and then counter rotated to affect the forward thrust downward.

It helps to gain the feel of this storage of energy in this strike if you visualize a strong rubber band stretching from the fingers of the left hand to the right hand.

With your right hand on top in holding the ball posture, rotate the ball one eight turn. As you store energy in the upward direction, do so with the feeling of stretching this rubber band. This will assist you in learning to store the energy of opening.

As in peng position, the events that are critical to timing are as follows in order of occurrence: initiate inhale; the first four of the nine pearls; beautiful lady's hand; opening; rotate the waist toward the rear foot and open the chest as you contract the diaphragm in "reverse Taoist breathing"; raise the hand to head height; compression of the muscles by torsion; balance is maintained over yong-chuan by pressing downward and lifting the hip with this motion; compression of the sacral pump, rotation of the waist away from the rear foot; breathe out; forward thrust of the hips as the hand is lowered in the direction of the candle with a shallow arc toward the tantien; and finally stop the hand.

11-2 Palm Strikes

The Palm strike differs from the others because an added component must be considered to gain the change of direction and a rotation of the palm (see figure 11).

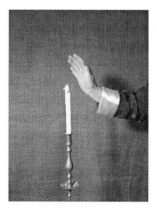

figure 11. Palm strike

The beginning of the cycle is the same as the peng position. The arc described by the hand on the emission cycle is a horizontal one, but it does not stop at the line drawn between the center of the practitioner and the opponent. It continues beyond this until it is stopped by the compression of the muscles of the right side.

This strike incorporates the jing of old ox power. The acceleration is begun by the rotation of the waist to the right, which bounces off the chan sichou of the right side and is delivered by a counter rotation to the left. With a right hand fa jin, it begins with a clockwise rotation of the waist in the emission cycle followed by a counterclockwise rotation after the body is turned to its farthest point to the right.

As the hips are thrust forward, the palm is rotated so it is facing forward. The strike is accomplished by using the xiao xing xing or small star of the palm. This is the area at the end of the arm bone, which is a continuation of a line drawn from the elbow through the center of the arm, up through the palm. It is as if the arm were a stick and the xiao xing xing was the tip of the stick or the end with which you would poke.

The palm must circumscribe a circle as it strikes. This circle is a large circle in training but becomes almost imperceptible when perfected. The strike must occur on the beginning of the upside of the circle to break someone's root, and on the downside when an jing is applied. This is a forceful, yet very short or abrupt circle that is at the end of the cycle and forms the release of qi.

An jing uses the tips of the fingers or the palm area or laogong point for the emission of energy. With the palm strike, it is important that you utilize the xiao xing xing area of the palm. This is the area that is directly in line with the long bones of the arm and will deliver the force of an jing without injury to the wrist caused by the hinge action of the hand and it will completely deliver the full force of the palm strike into the opponent.

The circles of the palm strike are the same as a strike from the peng position with the exception of a rotation of the palm on the forward thrust. This rotation allows the palm to face forward at the time of the strike. The circular rotation of the hand is counterclockwise as it is in peng, but included within this is the rotation of the palm forward. This excludes the use of the straightening of the beautiful lady's hand, but this is made up for in the loss of energy by the rotation of the forearm in conjunction with the palm rotation. It is more difficult to generate energy in the palm strike than the peng position because of this lack of energy developed in the beautiful lady's hand. It is, therefore, necessary to substitute this rotation of the forearm and to strike on the upward finishing circular stroke of palm strike to compensate for the loss of energy from the "beautiful lady's hand."

11-3 The Taiji Fist

The fa jin of Taiji utilized in a fist strike is in appearance one of a direct and short punch, which reveals little if any circular motion (see figure 12)

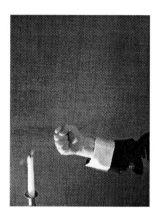

figure 12. Taiji fist

As with all other strikes of fa jin, the circles are there, though hidden within the subtlety of Taiji movement. Every movement within Taiji is circular. It is this deception that hides the real power and acceleration of motion that characterizes Taiji. It is only the distances that the hand moves along these arcs of the various circles that create the deception. All circles must be circumscribed in order to generate the power of fa jin. The linear appearance of the punch is only a deception created by the reduction of the distance moved on the outer circle.

The turning of the waist with little apparent movement of the hand gives the appearance of no power to the striking hand. It is nonthreatening to the opponent and may even be ignored by the unwary opponent. The lack of chambering also gives the sense that nothing is happening, so no counter is necessary.

The storage occurs with an almost imperceptible movement of the waist in a counterclockwise direction. This is along the horizontal circle with the tantien at its center and the hand on the arc of this circle. The hand is centered on the body and moves imperceptible with this centerline. The hand moves in minute circles in response to the movements of the body. There is a counter rotation in a clockwise direction when the waist is reversed. This circle of the hand is a shallow "S" shape. The hand then has a linear appearance as it approaches the target. It then makes a circular motion depending on the intended results, with the arm as the center of rotation or axis, and you want to uproot the opponent then strike the opponent on the upside of the circle. If you wish to drive the energy down into the ground and rebound, then you strike on the downward side of the circle. This circle as with the others in actuality is an imperceptible one. In practice however, it is necessary to begin with large circles and with success at the candle, shorten the circles to the point that they are imperceptible. There are many advantages to the Taiji punch. Punching from a balanced and stable root is one, another is the lack of chambering of the striking hand, but most important is the concealment of the forces within the circles of motion of the Taiji strike.

11-4 Filing Strike

This particular strike is a grazing strike. The forward motion of the edge of the knife hand is used as a strike to the body section with a component that moves the body in the direction of the strike (see figure 13).

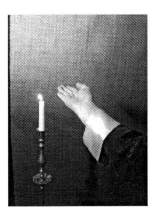

figure 13. Filing strike

For instance, a strike to the carotid sinus with a filing fa jin will result in a cavity strike and a forceful movement of the body backwards in the application of a technique to take the opponent down.

The application of this technique at the candle is only a variation in the point of contact with the body. The energy at the candle must be at the side of the candle and the direction parallel to the line from the tantien to the candle. The release of energy is from old ox power, which will have an energy component that is counterclockwise and therefore emits a force grazing the candle flame. In this configuration, the energy of compression is a at forty five-degree angle with respect to the horizontal plane

11-5 Tile hand Jab

This particular strike is not much different in the arcs performed from those of the chopping strike, except that they are much shallower and have the appearance of a straight line strike.

11-6 Striking from Single Whip

This Taiji posture and all others that lead to fa jin can be practiced at the candle by pre-positioning so that the movement within the form leads you directly to fa jin the candle flame. This is excellent practice, because it allows you to release the qi from the free flowing movement of the form. The practice can be from the whip end or the palm strike (see figure 14).

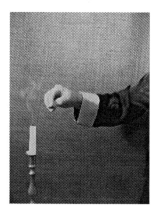

figure 14. Single whip

It is important to follow the movements of the form and distance yourself in front of the candle so that the correct movements can be made.

11-7 Secret Sword Hand

The secret sword hand was developed from battlefield conditions. The Chinese fought with two weapons, and they were equally skilled in both. If in the heat of battle, one weapon was lost, then the empty hand became the second weapon. The secret sword hand developed from this necessity (see figure 15).

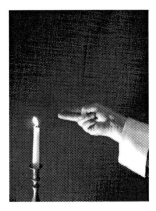

figure 15. Secret sword hand

This hand method consists of extending the first and second digits. The remaining digits are folded and the thumb is placed lightly over them.

11-8 One Finger Gong

One finger gong is the most difficult striking method to accomplish at the lazhu (see figure 16).

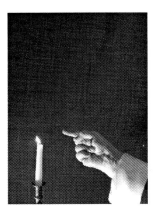

figure 16. One finger gong

This is due to the small striking surface. If you can fa jin with one finger gong then you are very accomplished. It requires considerable storage of energy and the complete release of all energies at the end of the cycle. More than any other striking method, it utilizes old ox power. Immense effort must be made to force the energy through the qi belt and the sacral pump. This is a straight thrust that requires all methods of energy storage to be impeccable.

11-9 Fatal Flute

If you can extend the qi to the tip of your weapon, then your open hand techniques will be considerably improved. The usage of the bamboo flute will greatly enhance your capabilities in the use of weapons as well as open hand techniques (see figure 17).

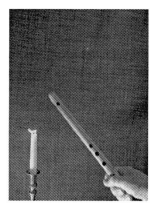

figure 17. Fatal flute

The flute then becomes a natural means of training within the weapon systems and can serve as a means of initiating weapons training.

The bamboo flute at the candle will train the student in relaxation techniques, which are extremely important in stick fighting. The speed required to use this weapon can only be attained with total relaxation. To be able to strike fast and with great power is required in this art form. The techniques for stick fighting, as far as extending the qi, are the same as empty hand techniques. The value in the flute at the candle is that it requires a considerable refinement of your techniques to be effective with the flute, and this can greatly enhance your empty hand techniques.

Section Four:
Higher Consciousness

12

Mind Body Relationship

12-1 Stilling the Mind

The usage of a specific form of meditation within an internal style of a martial art varies with the personal preference, or dictates of the specific internal art in question. What is constant is the central theme of the meditation. The central theme with respect to meditation is this constant effort to still the mind. What can be determined from these differing styles, internal and external, is this idea that is central to all styles. To still the mind removes the dichotomous thinking to which we are addicted. To dichotomize is literally to categorize things, place them into compartments, which have a limiting effect on our thinking. It places them into a yes-no, up-down hot-cold relationship. Part of this dichotomizing is the naming of the object. This places it in the "is or is not and this or that category," with names, actions and logical sequences which predetermine the course of our thinking. In the same manner, a mathematical equation leads us to a predetermined answer, so to does our logical thinking drive us to a conclusion based on our original premise. It is the premise that determines the logical conclusion. The sequencing of our own words builds the structure for our thinking. This is why po seems so alien to our natural way of thinking. The thought processes of po are imagery, visual representations, and are very symbolic in nature. The imagery has emotional attachments, which are a product of our experiences with the wisdom mind. It is important to realize that the emotions are of and by the wisdom mind and not a product of po. It is the intensity that po is interested in as this reflects only an energy level in the focus of po. Emotions are a product of past experiences and po operates within the eternal now and has no concept of past or future. Stilling the mind is no more than depriving oneself of the words by which the wisdom mind maintains its preeminence. Meditation is the constant attempt to deprive the wisdom mind of its stock in trade, words, by which it can manipulate and dominate the sensibilities of the observer shen. We do this by substituting visual imagery for the words of the wisdom mind. Visualization is the domain of po. All real and creative thinking is done on a visual imagery basis and then translated into the logical framework of the egomaniacal wisdom mind which then takes full credit for this and all other accomplishments. The more visual and less verbal you are, then the closer to po you become. It is not an act of totally removing the wisdom mind. This would put you totally within the realm of po. This is a totally foreign existence and not within the world of the ten thousand things. It is necessary to have one foot in each of the two worlds and their existence is then parallel and interactive. It is the nature of the wisdom mind to be active and the world of po is reactive (yang and yin). It is po that straddles these to worlds. By being in proximity of each other, there is a constant interaction. It is one in which the best of both worlds merge and the real you, as the observer, rapidly oscillate between these two worlds so that these appear as one, but they are in reality separate and distinct. The information is shared and processed in specific ways that accelerate the thinking process.

You are never more alive than when this condition exists. The whole body sings with the vibration of this oscillation. Thrill seekers strive for this. It is the exhilaration of sports, and it is the excitement that comes from quantum leaps of the thought processes. It is the rapid transfer of information and the commingling of knowledge and control. This mutual interlude is under the auspices of the wisdom mind, in that it delineates the direction of activities by means of desire, with its emotionally charged energy leading with the active principle hun and po reacting to the amount of energy contained within the imagery of hun only as a source of energy to be manipulated. It is through training techniques with visualization that we tie these two separate but cooperating entities together. It may not be fully understood, but imagery exists within hun and po. They share the imagery but not the emotional content. Emotion and desire are viewed merely as, high or low energy by po. It is the amount of energy that interests po. When we still the mind, we retain the imagery and retain the energy level. Po reacts to high energy level situations. Its interest is that of a small child. The glitter and sparkle of the situation interests it. This always reminds me of an old Abbot and Costello movie, in which Lou finds a bankroll of money and throws away the money and then plays with the rubber band in which it was wrapped. Hun would keep the money. It is po that throws away the money and plays with the rubber band.

The wisdom mind attempts to keep everything within its realm, that of the ten thousand things. It does this by intellectually assessing the problem. It is po that interacts with the problem. It is by sleeping on the problem that we solve it, and sleep is the domain of po. There is an ancient Taoist saying: "One light one dark is the way of the tao" This has been intellectualized to the maximum within the realm of the wisdom mind. There is great discussion of its meaning within the world of the ten thousand things. It is, however, within the domain of po that its meaning is evident. Po is the experiential realm. It is directly accessed and symbolic in its nature. The way is the direct experience of the one light and one dark. It is this experience that opens everything to be experienced rather than logically scrutinized. This is the experience of the void that is not empty followed by the golden light or chin hua.

The Book of Changes or I Ching is in reality a literary compilation of divination sources. Through the centuries, it has developed into an every day ritualistic divination about fate. Its original intent from its beginnings with the Ta Chuan or The Great Treatise was to determine whether the way was open or closed. It was a means of determining whether access to po and ultimately shen was open. Stilling the mind was a prerequisite to divination. Divination was the means to determine whether the way was open.

12-2 Withdrawal of the Senses

This is a method of meditation that restricts the input from the world of the ten thousand things. We cease to attend to those thoughts, ideas and sensations that would serve to keep us within the domain of the wisdom mind. The closer we get to po the more determined and active the wisdom mind becomes. It seeks preeminence and will do everything in its power to prevent po from becoming the dominant one in this duality. It is a way of determining how close you are to this mutual and parallel existence that is revealed by the active determined attempts of the wisdom mind to foil this attempt. The temple guard can become hysterical and all out of proportion to the situation. It has been likened by the ancient sages to a monkey leaping from tree to tree screaming at anyone within earshot. It seeks to toss idea after idea at the observer to captivate its attention and keep it within its domain. Withdrawing the senses does not involve forcefully removing yourself from the input of the senses, but instead is a relaxed effort to remove you from the phenomenal world and when it does impinge, to merely acknowledge it and contain it in a relaxed manner, to withdraw the senses. It is the reactive principle (yin in nature) that is pre-eminent and this is a shared existence. One only needs to acquiesce, acknowledge the momentary intrusion of the world of the ten thousand things, and move on. If too much effort is made to eliminate the offending thoughts, it places your efforts at a reduced sensory experience into an active ego-intensive effort of the yi mind.

12-3 Focusing the Mind

Many objects can be the focus of attention, and most of these are selected for meditation because they duplicate events on the road to enlightenment. For the purpose of Taiji, the focus should be on the opponent. He should be visualized while doing the form, even if this is only the sense of a presence. The opponent should be visualized in interception practice, and while doing the fighting sequence solo. The interception should be visualized at the candle and the strike should be aimed at the visualized opponent represented by the candle. The candle is only a representation of the opponent. The more you are effortlessly focused, the closer you are to po.

12-4 The Po

The continuity of existence we identitify as ourselves has been labeled by many as the spirit, observer, and the watcher, the ghost within the machine or deus ex machina, and po by the Chinese. This is what is left when we follow that classical imaginative game of eliminating the body segments and the sense's one by one, until all that is left, that is still you, is called the soul or shen. It is po that gives us access to shen and we arrive at shen through po. Usually, we go no farther than po, and we attain shen only with utmost difficulty.

The Chinese separate the tao into two categories, the undivided, Great One, into the dark (feminine spirit) which is yin, and the light (masculine spirit) which is yang. It is the interplay of these two forces when they separate from the tao that yields the ten thousand things or the natural phenomenal world. It is also the interplay between the forces of yin and yang that return the shen to the tao.

The Great One separates into these two natural forces, yin and yang, and following these forces form the dichotomies of kun and ch'ien. From yin the receptive feminine principle, kun is derived, and the masculine principle yang creates ch'ien. It is from these two natural forces that the human polarities are derived. kun and ch'ien are differentiations within yin and yang and are a part of them. The separation is a product of our dichotomous thinking and this separates man from the forces of nature.

Ming is organic and a natural aspect of life. Our existential fate is contained within its existence. It is not a realm of existence, which interacts, with the world of the ten thousand things. It lives a separate but parallel existence. If you can label it and assign meanings to it, then it is not ming. It exists beyond the world of words and logic. It is a world of energy and natural forces that do not resemble any description that has any relevance in the phenomenal world.

The essential nature of human existence is characterized by the principle xing. It emerges from of the yang aspect of the separation of tao. Xing contains the existence that is the entire world of the ten thousand things. Ten thousand to the ancient Chinese was an incredibly large number and it was used to describe the many manifest things of existence. It was a term that included all that we know, or can know.

It is out of these two disparate worlds of existence that hun and po come into existence. Hun is the knowable existence with which we are comfortable. It is our everyday existence and hun is the ego driven yi mind or wisdom mind that attempts to dominate this existence. Hun is the means by which we manipulate forces within the world of the ten thousand things or xing. Po is the means by which we manipulate forces within the realm of ming the physical body existence. There is a constant conflict between these two operating systems. It is an eternal ongoing battle for preeminence between these two disparate realms.

Hun is equipped with the greater resources and it is considered by the Chinese to be the active principle. Po is reactive and at a disadvantage. This leads to a predominance of hun in the interaction within the existence of xing and ming. Preeminence in this sense means only that the observer or shen exists within one or the other of these realms. Po can only operate within one of these worlds at a time and when it appears that it is operating in both, it is merely oscillating between the two so fast that it cannot be determined as a separate existence. It is this close proximity and rapid oscillation, which yield the vibrations that make us feel so alive at those moments when they are apparently working in unison, and this mind body relationship is at its peak. Po is the vehicle for the observer within its domain. It is not the actual spirit or ultimate essence of existence. This essence is the observer or shen.

For martial purposes, it is necessary to understand this mind-body relationship that exists within both realms. We know what it is to operate within the realm of hun. It is our everyday existence. Po, however, is an unknown, and because it is reactive, it is unresponsive unless it is trained. Po is very important within the internal martial sphere. It is reactive and the response is more precise and with greater speed than it would be within the realm of hun. Because of the greater range of its involvement, and the intricacies of its decision making process, hun is much slower than po. It is because of this, that po is trained to be pre-eminent when a fist interception is necessary. Much of the specifics of training that is so unusual in Taiji are for the purposes of accessing po. It is hun, however, that must train po, because only hun has access to past and future, and knows how to manipulate it. Po is only trained in patterns of behavior that do not require any concept of past or future. It only reacts to what exists at the moment.

12-5 The Vibrations

The martial interest in cultivation of and therefore access to po is because of the access to an expansive and manipulable source of qi, which can be used to supplement martial effort. Because po is reactive, it is necessary to utilize hun in coordination with it. This is because po operates within the eternal now and has no concept of past or future. The response is immediate and is in reaction to an immediate threat. This reaction occurs only due to prior training with specific purposes in mind. Logical reasoning does not prevail within the domain of po. It is for this reason that po and hun must operate in close proximity. It is hun, which through the logical aspects of its domain guides po in the utilization of the forces available only through this alternate domain. Without training and without the intercession of hun, po would be in a state of trance, much like a hypnotic trance. It would be unresponsive because it cannot interpret past or future consequences, therefore po cannot formulate a plan of action. It lacks the necessary logical tools and the ability to manipulate words. Often what occurs when we are attacked and we do nothing and are completely unresponsive, we are merely immediately in the unfearing domain of po? It is the excessive fear that causes hun to escape the immediate threat and dump the problem on an unprepared po. Hun is the coward and will bail out of an extreme situation in an instant. Unfortunately, what is usually left is an untrained po, totally incapable of an appropriate response.

It is necessary to train po in the appropriate behavior when confronted by a threat. It is impossible to train po in the means of determining a threat in the conventional sense. It is necessary to predetermine some triggering events that are part of the threat and use these in a manner that will facilitate an immediate access to po. One of those elements that can be used as triggering devices is the fact that the closer we get in proximity between po and hun, some very specific things begin to occur within the body. The spirit or shen, which is also called the observer that exists within you, begins to shift perspective. It oscillates between po and hun at a rapid pace. The higher the frequency of this vibrational shift, then the closer the two are. The more the two are in synch, then the more receptive po is to dictates of the hun on a visual basis.

This coordination between hun and po cannot be done within the realm of the logical mind. It must be done nonverbally, in a symbolic language of visualization or sensory learning. The most effective training is through visualization, but there are times of greater capability. If this state of heightened frequency of oscillation can be attained during training, then it is more effective.

We often have this feeling of excitement, in which it seems our body is charged with electricity and our performance is at its peak. What we are experiencing is this rapid oscillation or vibration between po and hun. It is during this stage of heightened interaction, in which hun is in a sense directing po, that the yi mind can lead po, with its collaboration, down a specific training experience. It is this mutual cooperation of the logical past and present operation of hun in cooperation with po's forces of qi and direct access to body responses that accelerate the martial response. This is yi yi yin qi.

It would seem that increasing this feeling of rapid oscillation during training sessions would accelerate the close approximation of hun and po. An interesting note to all this is that this experience in some people can lead to what they would consider pathology. Many people go to physicians with complaints of tinnitus, which is a ringing sensation in the ears. Often this is no more than the vibrational oscillations of po and hun. This sensation can be a key to determining the accessability of po. It can be used to determine the effectiveness of our attempts at accessing po. We can cultivate those efforts that lead to this vibration. The Chinese call this ringing the dragon's hum and the tigers roar. The dragon's hum occurs in the left ear and the tiger's roar occurs in the right ear. The existence of the dragons hum and the tiger's roar indicate that training can be effective at that time. The difference between tinnitis and the dragon's hum and tigers roar is the constancy of the vibrations. Dragons hum and tigers roar will ebb and flow with the accessability of po. Tinnitis will be constant.

12-6 Po in Two Worlds

The worlds of po and hun never merge. They are parallel in their existence, but they do not merge with each another. There is a devious coordination for mutual benefit. Both seek preeminence in their determined effort at access to the physical body. In that respect, po is unique in that it can operate not only indirectly within the realm of the ten thousand things, but it can operate in the world of shen. Po is the interface between the physical world and the world of spirit or shen. It is because of this dual operational capacity that po is able to manipulate the forces of both worlds. It is not entirely accurate to express it in this manner. The true existential reality and the essence of existence are not characterized by po. It is the observer that oscillates between po and hun. The two are no more than operating systems, each with their own respective capabilities and operating environments. It is zhenzheng ren or the observer, the immortal or genuine person, who uses these systems each in turn with their limitations. These two systems combined by this oscillating feature can be formidable. These two systems operate and have an existence that is ongoing and separate from shen, but it is shen that is the reality, or the existence of the observer within shen. shen is awareness.

The body has its own maintenance system that keeps it operating independent of the location of shen. Each of the two operating systems is struggling for the capture of shen, the observer. It is the conscious identity that we experience, as ourselves. Shen is awareness that looks out on the world with a formidable curiosity.

It is po that can view shen in its natural environment. It views shen indirectly by viewing the energy forms that pour in from the world of shen into the physical body through various portals in the human body. Remember it is the energy of the body and the spirit that is the domain of po. It manipulates the energy system of the body and also regulates the infusion of energy from the tao

A simple test of your ability to access po and indirectly view shen requires no more than the placement of your attention on the bai hui. If you look straight forward at the horizon, then the top most portion of your head is the bai hui. When you place your attention on the bai hui (hundred meetings), it is important that you do not place any intent or desire on the crown center. You must look at it from the side. You must be aware of it, but not interact with it or attempt any thing with intent or any action (wu wei). It should be understood that any attempt is a feature of the yi mind and will divert you into its domain. You must access po and remain within po for a considerable time. This is a waiting without intent and by looking askance you maintain your attention on the bai hui.

If you can do this properly and for a considerable period of time, then you will experience a sensation of something wiggling out of the crown center. This is the opening of the bai hui. If you can accomplish this for enough time and repeat it an innumerable number of times, you will eventually be a witness to the forces of energy pouring into the body at the bai hui energy gate.

12-7 Breathing and the Mind Body Relationship

It is by means of the natural process of breathing that we can learn to control po. By directly controlling breathing, we can indirectly control po. The physical processe of the body is the domain of po. There is a reciprocal relationship between the various bodily processes. Heart rate and breathing rate are intertwined for survival purposes. If we can increase or decrease one, we can alter the other. It is possible for us to regulate and control the breathing and in so doing we can alter the heart rate. If we can regulate heart rate then we can control our state of mind and eliminate fear and emotion from any encounter. This is our means of access to the autonomic system, which is not under the direct control of the wisdom mind, but can be indirectly controlled.

12-8 The Art of Flying

Probably the most effective way of initially accessing po is through visualizing flying while in the dream state. This is so because it utilizes many different methods that are anathema to the preeminence of hun. Animism is characteristic of the shamanistic traditions and those similar in ritual. Flying is not simply a method of assuming the characteristics of the animal or bird, although this does facilitate what is attempted, but it is instead a mental transformation or a visualization of your as the animal. This is necessary in order to move throughout the world of po. Just as the fear of flying can project you beyond the world of the ten thousand things, so too can this transformation or visualization take you beyond this world. The rational mind does not accept this leap into the irrational. The more that the practitioner can assume the animal as himself; the closer to po he is operating. To meet someone within the realm of po is to stalk them with the animal persona, not in a violent way but in a way of animal curiosity. The practitioner becomes the predator within the realm of po and moves throughout his domain with this reality firmly in grasp. Many of the animal styles are misunderstood and are interpreted as simply imitations of the animals fighting behavior. In the shamanistic tradition, you are the animal: you have become the personification of the animal. This animism is controlled by the desires and intentions of the wisdom mind. There is no feedback within the realm of po. Therefore, even if you are successful in completely immersing yourself with po, there is no corroboration of ongoing activities without the feedback from another participant, or else a close cooperation with the yi mind. It is like leaping off into the abyss where the act itself results in the reality within po because the rational mind cannot deal with contradictions to the yi mind's self-appointed authoritarian logic. If it defies rationality, then hun rejects it or escapes from it. It is our intention to force hun to escape from this aberrant behavior and allow po to ascend by this leap into the abyss in a dreamscape. Yes it is true that it helps to be a little bit crazy.

13

The Nature of Po

13-1 Ineffability of Po

One of the most intriguing aspects of po is the absence of feedback, which will give some semblance of causality. The appearance of a non-causal relationship is one of the things happening to you without your ego-direct access or control. As the observer, there exists this disconnect and it exists between you as the performer and the performance itself. To further, confound the situation, while in the realm of po there is no linear sequencing of thought, which is evident with the use of words. It is a linguistic requirement that words are strung sequentially and in proper order. There is no such requirement with symbolic thought. Symbols are always comprehended in the totality of the situation and are perceived as being immediate and non-sequential. The symbolic and the real are often confounded when operating in the domain of po. The symbolic and real are seen as having equal weight and each in terms of po are dealt with as if they were in fact real.

13-2 Po and the Golden Flower

The Golden Flower or Chin Hua occurs with the interplay of hun and po. It is the result of this interaction between these disparate modes of existence that the Golden Flower occurs. It is from this oscillation between these two modes in close proximity that separation of the observer from hun to po can occur. This allows a view of the spirit or shen world from the vantage point of po. Both worlds can be viewed at once. It is possible for po to ascertain both worlds at once, but from an observational point of view only. This requires a separation of the observer from the physical body. This is a separation from the body to a point of near proximity to the body. Without this close proximity, there is a loss of memory.

This separation from the physical body occurs when po withdraws from the body and the proximity of hun is decreased. As the distance increases, the oscillation of po decreases in frequency so that the observer actually senses existence first in hun and then in po and not as if existing in both simultaneously. Existence, as a point in space, becomes one of the material worlds looking toward po and the next second within po looking back toward hun or yiwan dongxi. This translocation continues until a distance of a few feet. Beside the altering viewpoint, there is a sensory experience in this separation. This separation is felt as if the filamental attachments at the juncture of the body were being withdrawn and the sensation is as if a thin thread were being drawn across these points at each point of attachment. It is interesting to note that these connection points are along a lateral line denoting front and back halves of the body. This is comparable to the lateral line in fish, which is a line of electrical activity and sensory capabilities.

This is a slow transition from hun to po and is not necessarily the way it will usually occur. The slow process is one of a learning sequence in which the individual is presented with a sensory experience that depicts this transition as a progression of events. There are structural visualizations that accompany this separation and they indicate the existence of something within the realm of po that is a connection, and it is a part of po. The connection is from po to hun and not the reverse. It would seem from this that the real existence of the true self is extending from the tao through shen and then to po and finally to hun and the existence of the temporal body.

13-3 The World of Po

Existence within the state of po can be alluded to by those states, which we can identify as contrary to existence within the wisdom mind or hun. We have already described some states that would indicate a contradistinction. We know that dreaming of flying or standing at levels above, certain heights are not conducive to the state of hun. If we can describe the conditions of these states, it may lend some degree of comparison to hun. The ususal tendency is to describe it in terms of this-not this. When you use the world of the ten thousand things as a basis for comparison, then everything is going to be "not this" with respect to po. It then becomes a matter of describing what it does rather than what it is. If you describe po in terms of what it does, then you are describing its interaction with the energy system of the body. Access to and utilization of the energy system is through po, so any description of this interaction can lead to an understanding of what po is.

It is po's responsibility to maintain a balance within the energy system of various parts of the body. All post-natal qi enters the body from outside through the realm of po. It is channeled to the body through the various energy locations (chakras), and then distributed through the channels and meridians. We also know that if something is done seemingly without our doing it (wei wu-wei), then it probably is po that is pre-eminent. Any of the various trance states would be within the realm of po unless we are accessing verbal centers.

13-4 The Form and Po

There is much to be said for the proper way to do the form. There is even more reason for doing it wrong. This is not a contradiction. To say that the proper way to do the Taiji form is to do it incorrectly means that if you do have problems staying within the proper sequence of the form after years of practice, it only means that you are treading that fine line between po and the wisdom mind (hun). This is not an intellectual exercise in which you can answer the questions academically and you pass. To do the form properly, is to place po and hun in close proximity and test continually whether it is po or hun that is pre-eminent. This is not something intentional, but is instead a function of the way in which you do the form. If you are operating within hun and you perceive the world of the ten thousand things then it is hun that is pre-eminent. In order to do the form properly, you must still the mind, have the sense of the opponent before you, and think only of the next posture in the sequence of the form. Po is stressed in doing the form because we normally operate within the wisdom mind. It is proper to lead po with the wisdom mind, but it is only by the occasional lapse in performing the sequence that we know we have escaped within po. Remember it is po that operates within the eternal now, and if you can contain your thoughts within the immediate form in a visual sense with only an occasional slip into words, then you are scalloping between the two worlds and they are in close proximity.

It is axiomatic that the better you do the form for martial purposes, then the more you will do it in error. The form is a training tool for the martial purposes of training po in the procedures and tactics of the martial arena. The error that occurs within the form is this disconnect between po and the wisdom mind. When you are operating only within po, then you lack the direction of the wisdom mind and po wanders in search of energy. This is similar to scalloping in sailing. In order to know how close you are to the wind, you must oscillate between luffing and stalling the sail periodically to determine your best position.

If you lose yourself in the form, it is that you have lost the proximity of po and the yi mind. The remedy is to test yourself periodically or determine key points that will signal your location within the form. The form can be broken into various segments from one single whip form to the next. You can test the wind at this point and see where you are in the form, without losing this proximity of po and yi.

13-5 The Spirit of Po

To operate within the realm of po is to be disconnected or disembodied. It is this lack of awareness of the physical existence, due primarily to the absence of sensory feedback that characterizes po. If there is a sense of the body being moved without any effort on your part, then you are observationally within hun and operationally within po. This oscillation is one of observation within the world of the ten thousand things and activity within the world of po. The fact that we can do many things at one time comes as no surprise. What is surprising is the fact that, we can also operate within a realm in which we are unaware of causation, yet can be aware of the results.

13-6 The Plasma Body

The energy that exists within po is the plasma body, so called because of its appearance as a glowing high-energy gaseous candle flame-like covering of the body. It is evident only in the dark of night because of its very close proximity to the body, and the faintness of its light. It glows with the effervescence of a gaseous or liquid golden shimmer that resides within inches of the body. It is energy that is tied to the body. It is a result of the functioning of these bodily processes, and it can only be seen by others when they are within the state of po. It does not fall within the visible spectrum that can be seen by the yi mind.

There are various stages that will be seen when viewing the plasma body. These are artificially selected stages that demarcate points of interest. What actually happens is that the view of the plasma image goes from one of high intensity to one of diminished intensity. It is during the diminished portion that structural things become evident. The incident can occur for instance when you are aroused from a very deep sleep in the early hours of the morning (huo banye). You are not quite awake and probably deep within po and on the verge of access to the yi mind. If you are fortunate, you will see in someone else a liquid light pouring down from the bai hui point filling the body from the top down with a golden phosphorescent light. As it descends, the demarcation line will take on the appearance of a drape as it follows the curvature of the body until it is totally encompassed by this ethereal light.

There will be a gradual diminishment in the intensity of the glow and eventually it will be apparent that the body is uniformly covered with points of greater intensity. These points of greater intensity appear to be nodules or conical elevations from deeper within and formed on the lower layer and they are projected to near the top surface. The spaces between the nodules seem to be filled with light of a lesser intensity from orange to a brown glow. The brighter portions of the nodules seem to be filled with filaments pouring energy into the phosphorescent layer of light.

The relevance of the ephemeral light is that it is within the depths of po that access to this energy of hua jing will occur. The deeper you are within po means, then the closer you are to a trance like state and farther from this interactive state between yi and po that is necessary for martial purposes. There are ways that you can access this energy and use it for martial purposes. It will be difficult to access po to the depths of its existence since it is a trance like state and the greater the depth then the farther you are from the ten thousand things and your accepted reality. Fear may keep you from this deep access.

14

The Mystery of Shen

14-1 The Immortal

Zhen zheng ren is the Chinese term for an immortal. The Chinese considered one who breathes through his heels as an immortal. This is a reference to the practice of qi gong, in which visualization of breathing from the heel through the body to the fingertips and then releasing the qi at the fingertips can eventually lead to enlightenment. An enlightened individual is considered an immortal. It is through reversing the flow of qi in the universal orbit that enlightenment can occur.

Immortality is considered possible by those that have transformed themselves into shen. The normal spirit of the average individual is called kuei, which translates as ghost being. It hovers in the area of death and is a dark being. Its existence eventually ceases some time after death.

The existence of the sage is far different from that of the normal individual. Most immortals do not associate with the human community. There are some that do and their purpose is the elevation of humanity and that of bringing all of humanity into this sage condition.

14-2 The Secret Chamber

Within the area behind the brow, is the pineal gland. This esoteric feature is often called the third eye because it is made up of photosensitive cells. Past research has revealed that each living cell emits a pulsing light. All cells of the same type beat in unison, and this is a natural process of communication between cells. The research consisted of placing cells in a glass Petrie dish culture medium and then positioning another similar culture next to it. When a substance was added to one dish destroying the cells, those in the adjacent dish also were affected, and they died. It was discovered by using quartz dishes, which will not transmit ultraviolet rays, that the ultraviolet rays were the method of communication. This indicates how important light is to the communication of cells.

The pineal gland functions in a communication network in the realm of po. It is the interface between the world of po and the ten thousand things. It is through the secret chamber that po can look backward toward the body and at the same time look forward into the shen (see figure 18). It is not possible to describe this world in a measurable scientific sense, but it is possible to elaborate on the perceptual truths that are evident within po. Much of science is the indirect measurement of events. It is this lack of measurement that makes qi so elusive, but there are consistent descriptions that have not changed cross-culturally or over time. These are very good indications that something exists perceptually consistent and uniform within the realm of human nature (xing) that is of paramount importance to the human condition.

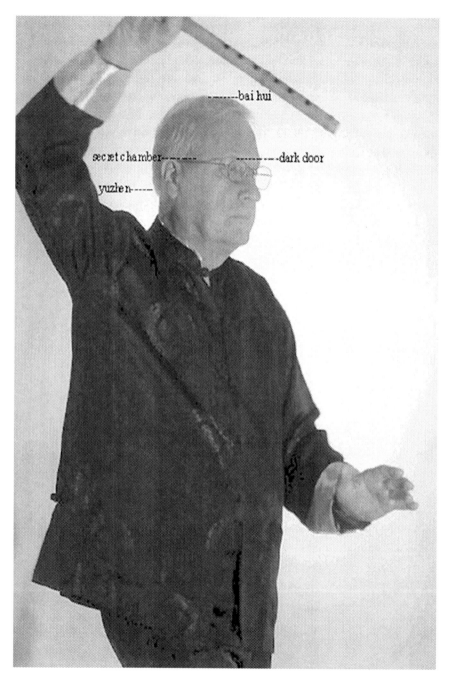

figure 18. The Secret Chamber

The secret chamber is entered by various combinations of methods. Meditating on this center can sometimes yield access. Reversing the flow of qi so that it flows up the spine and into the secret chamber is another. It is through this route that the martial arts have become a means of attaining enlightenment. It is common for internal martial artist to regulate the flow of qi in this manner. They reverse the normal flow to that of a flow from the foot to the extended hand. The only difference is that in meditation the energy flow is extended up through the neck, the head and across the skull into the secret chamber. Martial arts training can be a preliminary to the final meditation leading to and becoming an immortal, in the Chinese sense of the word, which means enlightened.

14-3 The Reverse Flow of Qi

This is the method of reversing the flow of qi within the small universe circulation or xiao chou tien. The normal flow of qi is from the tantien through the hui yin up the back past the ming men to the crown point or bai hui and down the front side to return to the tantien. What happens in the practice of fa jin is that this process of delivering qi to the fingertips is a short-circuiting of this reversal or xiao cho tien. It is because of this apparent reversal in fa jin that Taiji is considered a walking meditation. The potential for long-term training in the reversal of flow of the qi is readily apparent.

14-4 The Meaning of Life

The single most important activity that you can do to elevate your level of consciousness is to question your relationship with the Tao. You must have an interest in this relationship and seek out solutions to the perplexing problems presented by this search. It is not that any specific answers will be forth coming, but rather that in an experiential sense the answers will be revealed, and these answers will be in the form of an interactive relationship between Heaven and Earth, with Humanity at its center. It is expected that answers will be forthcoming within the logical framework of the rational mind. These answers (those of the meaning of life), however, are revealed by a symbolic representation, a revelation of process, and not structure. We experience the visualizations as a genuine real process in life.

14-5 Yi Yi Yin Qi

It is by means of the yi mind leading the qi through predetermined routes within the body that martial techniques occur. Yi yi yin qi is a common statement within the Taiji community. To understand this concept, you must have an appreciation for what occurs within the body during visualizations.

We can begin with what happens as we learn to read. The first thing we learn is the letter "A." Our eye traces the letter and memorizes its geometrical outline. As we learn to write the letter first by tracing its outline and then by repetitive copies on paper, we are memorizing the minute muscular contractions that our whole body makes in transcribing the letter, it is this combination of eye and body movements that we memorize. When we remember the letter "A," it is these minute contractions we recall and duplicate. On some level, we are always making all the detailed movements that accompany this memorization process.

When we practice at the lazhu, we begin with large circles and reduce them eventually to almost imperceptible movements. This is not the end of it. This is the beginning of yi yi yin qi. It is by visualizing every detail of the strike without movement that we create the minute muscular contractions that initiate the flow of qi. Our practice at the lazhu then becomes one of primarily visualizations and reduced effort at extinguishing the lazhu.

14-6 Tai Yi Jin Hua Congshi

This is translates as the secret of the golden flower. This is enlightenment or the intensification of awareness. This does not mean just ordinary sensory awarness, but more importantly awareness in the realm of kun. It is from our existential confrontations that we develop this increased self-awareness, but also with enlightenment, we enter into the arena of po and thereby enter this esoteric world that encompasses our existence. It does not present you with the gift of sainthood or even make you better person. What it does is shift your awareness and perspective as to your relative importance within the Tao. It creates a feeling of being immersed within the Tao and you become a part of the natural order of things.

There unquestionably are some important advantages to enlightenment, in the same sense that color vision gives a slight advantage to the individual. This advantage occurs over the millennia and as an individual; these slight differences may not be significant. As a species, we have evolved and continue to evolve. Even as an individual, we evolve from a single cell up through the various stages of life. Past successes as a species are indicators of future potential. Everything in existence is in a state of change bordering on chaos. As a species, we are in a state of constant flux.

The real secret within the secret of the golden flower is that there is an effervescent golden light within us that is a part of the immutable existence of this nugget of awareness we identify as self. All else is the proverbial illusion. This awareness is the reality and it becomes manifest in many ways throughout life.

14-7 The Tao

The tao exists and this existence cannot be defined. It is indescribable in everyday terms and can only be labeled in the realm of the of the logical wisdom mind. It is an existence that goes beyond the yin and yang classification or labeling of dichotomous thought. The very essence of naming it moves it into the existential category of something other than the tao. We think that by naming something, we have acquired some profound knowledge and understanding of the intimate nature of reality. This is merely substituting labeling and name recognition for true knowledge. The essential truth about the tao is that there is no truth about the tao. We have satisfied our desire for knowledge with simple name recognition. We feel that if we can name it then it can be intellectually manipulated and we have accomplished something important.

15

The Po

15-1 Be Like the Willow

The capability of flexing or being limber is the willow's essence. It quietly reforms itself with the forces of nature and offers no resistance that will take it past its breaking point. Taiji has the willow's same yielding unbreakable nature. Be like the willow is a common expression in Taiji. It is more than just offering little resistance to the forces being applied by the opponent. You also have the capability of using this yielding nature to redirect those incoming forces. It is beyond being nonaggressive and and offering no resistance, but instead it is this snap back capability of the willow. The inner resilience that allows the willow to return to its original position when these forces are no longer bending it is the nature and the strength of the willow. It is like the feather, wafting in the wind, unresisting and moving by something other than its own effort. It bends and to external forces and when they no longer exist, it snaps back as if they had never occurred. Undoubtedly, the most feared device within the childhood of most of us is the willow switch. With very little effort, it can inflict considerable pain. Most young children would rather take a beating than be confronted by the willow.

It is through this ability to deliver an accelerating sine wave to the tip that Taiji is compared to the willow. Just as it yields to the incoming forces, the very nature of its ability to return to its original position gives it the springiness that can accelerate forces to its tip. To be song is to be like the willow, non-resistant and yet having the ability to maintain position and return to the original position without the use of force.

It is this willow-like ability to stand in the face of forces with a serene detachment that characterizes po. It is the very essence of po. As with many things within Taiji, visualizations are a part of the training. In accessing po, if we visualize ourselves as if we were the willow, we then take on the attributes of the willow by moving and swaying with the forces of nature. With time, we discover that if we are like the willow, we are not within the realm of the yi mind, but have accessed po. Meditation and other techniques are mimicked by this visualization. You will find it is more direct and easier to maintain than meditation itself. So, be like the willow and you will be song.

15-2 Visualizations at the Candle

The possibilities of visualizations at the candle are enormous. Some of the more important ones include the sense of the enemy, movement of qi from the finger-tips through the body to the rear heel. The reverse flow of qi from the heel back to the fingertips on fa jin, the taiji ball, taiji sphere and moving the body as a whole should also be included.

All visualizations at the candle should be tied to fa jin. This allows us to make the connection of all visualizations with fa jin.

15-3 Visualizations of the Willow

The Willow is characterized by its capability of yielding to the onslaught of over-whelming force. This is contrary to our natural tendencies. We do not ordinarily tend to think that a tremendous force can be created by a yielding force. When we visualize the willow and its great flexibility while we fa jin with success we are then bolstering our concept that the soft can overcome the hard. We must imbue our visualizations with a sense of the various ways of generating force from yield-ing and soft techniques. These techniques will then eventually be incorporated into our everyday existence and become a part of our internal art.

15-4 Intuitive Practice of Perceiving the Attack

There are some general principles that assist in the overall perception of an attack. First, if your training is correct then your perception will be centered on the peripheral and not focused on the ten thousand things. There are specific stylized behaviors that occur in an attacker. These can be readily identified if you know some specifics about behavior that are visible but not obvious. Without getting into the technical aspects of behavior, there are some constants that occur when we become devious, duplicitous or subversive.

If the attacker is trying to get in close, then his attempt at deception is his undoing. When we are genuine and straight forward, we move straight forward, eyes and body centered openly on the individual of our intent. If his intent is not straight forward and open, then there are two alternatives. He can be pensive and be searching for information or be thoughtful in his approach. In this case, his body, eyes and head will be slightly and sometimes even exaggeratedly off center to the left. When we are searching for objective memory, we are searching specific memory areas in the brain. If we are thoughtful and not devious, we are centered to the left. If we are intent on ill will then we are off center to the right because our memory is processed through entirely different parts of the brain, those parts used for duplicitous memory as opposed to objective memory.

This is type of activity is quite noticeable when interrogating someone and they are searching their memory for an answer. If they are being evasive, their eyes will quickly dart to their right and then return to the center. When they are not being evasive and they are searching memory for an answer to a question their eyes will dart to their left and return to center. This is a guide for those who conduct interrogation. The value of this for the internal martial artist is that the first sign would be a movement of the individual toward us with his eyes and body slightly off center to their right.

There are other indications, which can be a sign that someone is surreptitiously attempting to close the distance and gain proximity to you. When a person is evasive, his movements become deliberate and stylized. This is due to nature of our processing complex information, rather than straight forward objective and unprocessed information.

In the same manner in which you trained with the swinging ball to create the trigger that would allow immediate access to po, you must train for these subtle cues that will also allow immediate access to po. It is more practical to view the perception of their orientation from your perspective. If they glance to the left, they are searching objective memory, and the body is oriented off center to their left, then from your perspective they are oriented off center to your right. Think of this as to your right is good and to your left is bad. Training would consist of movement of a partner toward you with each orientation, right or left of center with the simulated attack occurring when the opponent's orientation is to your left. At the candle, you can utilize visualization of an approaching attack with the orientation to your left, which should initiate po only if there is a perceived threat, but in training, we are training po in what we wish it to attend.

We can link the approach and the stylized chambering of the fist and develop a strategy that causes access to po even prior to the chambering of the fist. This accelerates the process increasing our advantage.

15-5 Tiao Xin Regulating the Emotional Mind

Tiao xin is initiated with stopping the internal dialogue using qi gong methods that still the mind and it results in the removal of all sequential and logical thought. A prerequisite to regulating the mind is to remove all thought first and then the thought of no thought will be preeminent. It is necessary to obviate the xin mind or emotional mind because the energy that is required for maintaining the yi mind and its preeminence is created by the xin mind or emotional mind.

The form is one of the most effective ways of controlling the xin mind. It is performed in a slow methodical way partially to regulate the xin mind. There are many other reasons, but the slowness of the form reflects the time distortions that occur when po is preeminent. The time distortions that typify po are present within the form and tend to lead the mind in the direction of po. Many of the meditation techniques are a mimic of conditions of the po mind as evidenced by mandalas and repetitious and stylized behavior within shamanistic practices. Regulating the xin mind is another means of diverting our mental preeminence from the yi mind.

15-6 Nei Shi Gong Fu

This has been defined as internal perception gong fu. It is through long practice that you develop the capability to deliver qi to the organs and muscles of the body at your choosing. It is also called the gong fu of internal vision because it is by virtue of visualizations and access to po that you can accomplish this.

15-7 The Mechanics of Accessing Po

One simple method of training for access to po is to use a sphygmomanometer (blood pressure monitor) and to use the reduction of blood pressure and pulse as an indicator of the presence of po. The rationale for this is the fact that most elevated blood pressure when we are resting is due to egocentric stresses from the social environment. The reduction of blood pressure has a health benefit that is incidental to accessing po, but gives us added incentive to try this method. The fact that we can reduce blood pressure by entering into this state of existence can be conducive to maintaining a lower blood pressure.

The pressure elevation is due to our being trapped in this fight or flight syndrome caused by the ego mind in its incessant attempt at preeminence. It is the assertiveness of the ego-mind; not only within its own physical body, but in the external environment and social environment as well that creates this conflict. The body resources are wasted on maintaining the artifice of the predominance of the ego-mind. In Taoist philosophy, it is the original mind that has preeminence and it is by virtue of the secret of the Golden Flower that we return to this natural preeminence of the Original Mind.

Accessing po, which stands between the yi mind and the Original Mind is accomplished by mimicking the conditions present in the state of the Original Mind. We calm the mind and eliminate desire and intent. This is done by following the breath. There is a slight of hand here that should be elaborated on, to make this access to po more understandable. We know that by creating conditions antithetical to the preeminence of the yi mind, such as boring repetitive actions the ego mind will escape the situation. We also know that visualizations will allow us access to po. We also know that we can set up a trip wire visualization that will allow access to po when attacked. The form, visualization at the candle and the interception visualization all contribute to gaining access to po. As we move in training from ming jing (visible force) to an jing (hidden force) and then finally to hua jing (perfect force), we are reducing the chambering and striking movement and increasing the visualization of the moving force in fa jin.

The visualizations, when applied directly to a combat situation can be very effective, but a word of warning is in order. As you increase your effectiveness at visualization through practice, you may become so adept at it that it can slip over into every day thought. It can be difficult sometimes to distinguish the reality of the moment, not necessarily in discriminating the reality, but that your body can and will react to visualizations just the same as if it were real. We can take advantage of this in training, but it also can adversely affect your body. The fight and flight reaction can be triggered if these visualizations are not in the realm of po. It is the absence of emotional content in po that keeps you from destroying your body with constant fight or flight reactions.

It is the cool slender breath that is the key to maintaining visualizations within po and not within yi.

15-8 Understanding the Training

Training is not conventional in the sense that you are attempting to improve your physical performance or even your mental performance. It is instead a constant attempt to promote, refine and deliver a coordinated action that comprises a mutual effort between po and the yi mind. If we are totally within the realm of the yi mind, then we do not have access to the vast and powerful forces inherent within the domain of po. If we are completely within the realm of po then we have vast resources of power and can interact with the scope of incoming and out going energies, but we do not have a sense of past or future consequences that can develop a plan, a solution or a means of even interpreting the situation within a social or psychosocial manner. We are in a sense an idiot savant. It is only when you operate within close proximity and can exchange information from one mode to the other that training makes any sense, so when we say we are training the mind it is not in the usual sense of mental training that we mean mental training.

It is the training of the mind that differentiates Taiji from other martial arts. It is mind against mind that drives the Taiji agenda. If you relinquish strength against strength, then all that is left is mind against mind or mind against strength. All the training is an attempt to convince the novice that these things are possible, because nothing happens if you do not accept the premises in the first place.

We can use simple devices to convince the mind that these things are possible and we can use methods of tricking the mind into accepting these premises. One method employed by the shamanistic traditions is to set up a journey with the apprentice with the warning that you must use death as your advisor. It is imperative that you do not look to your left since death will tap you on your left shoulder. It is not a good idea to look death in the face. You must always look to the right when you feel the approach of death. This sets up expectations making it extremely difficult not to look left. The mind of the apprentice is always on the left in an attempt to avert gazing left. The reason that this is effective has to do with the differences in memory access. There are interrogation methods in use that utilize the differences in memory access. It is known that when we are being duplicitous or evasive we access different areas of the brain than when we are simply accessing memory in an objective manner. If we are deceptive when asked a question, our eyes will dart to the right side of our body and to the left when we are simply searching for information. This has some relevance for Taiji training in that if you can set up conditions that are mentally conducive to accessing the intuitive areas of the brain rather than the devious and duplicitous areas, which are ego, functions and then we are closer to po.

One training method that can be used, which serves to exemplify this, is that the students can be trained to expect an arbitrary punch at any time during class. This sets up the expectation and their mind is constantly on the possibility. This expectation has the effect of training them to be receptive to the visualization practices that are used in interception practice. This helps in placing their mind closer to po than the yi mind, while it also serves to set up expectations of a specific behavior. It is not necessary to use repetitive practice in actual training if you can train with visualizations. It is in essence setting up the condition where the mind is tapping into memory of previous training, which is objective in nature, and not of the duplicitous ego functioning kind. This assures us that the effect of these simple expectations is training po and not the yi mind.

The Taoist tradition is to use natural methods rather than the interventionist methods of the Buddhists and external traditions. It is the use of the natural expectations of the individual that are effective. We take the individual as he exists within nature and use his natural tendencies. The training of the Taoist is in many instances so subtle that it does not appear as if it is training.

In training lazhu fangfa, we are moving through a series of stages that appear to be training something else instead of the movement of qi through the body to be expressed at the fingertips. It at first seems to be extremely mechanical and that it is a muscular, although an extremely subtle one that is being trained. It helps to understand that research within the Chinese qi gong community reveals that the delivery of qi seems to resemble the release of a sound wave in a pulse form that serves as a carrier wave to the delivery of qi. The mechanical and muscular portion of this training is that of learning to produce this carrier wave that can deliver the qi to the opponent in a martial sense and to the sick person in a healing environment. The level of performance is equally balanced between training the mind and coordinating the body so that all things are possible and that active intervention is at a minimum.

15-9 Techniques for Accessing Po

There are ten separate distinctions that can be made in the application of most techniques, they are as follows:

1. Connect	4. Stick	7. Seal	10. Push
2. Listen	5. Follow	8. Unbalance	
3. Adhere	6. Neutralize	9. Uproot	

Each one of these individual aspects of the technique can and should be used to train in accessing po. Connect is trained at the intercept of the soft ball through the means of visualization. With each intercept, the opponent should be visualized as if making the triggering movements that characterize the punch, grab or stab. It is important to remember that it is the visualizations that tie this all together and make it one complete whole. Listening can be trained with coiling techniques where the attempt at touching the forehead and abdomen serves as a means of training your ability to recognize the opponent's energy and your energy. This allows you to sense their intent. Stick is a more difficult concept to train within po. The difficulty lies in the fact that this must be trained within the yi mind and some how transferred to po. The simplest way to do this is to train visually in this along with actual practice. Visualization of the actual technique with emphasis on sealing techniques can be helpful. Follow can be trained at the ball by simply keeping your hand on your center as you follow the ball. If you maintain your center, then it will be necessary to move your waist in order to follow the ball. Neutralizing also can be trained at the ball by simply attempting to stop the ball with the back of your hand and thereby not allowing it to return, each technique should be used to seek out that particular aspect that illustrates each principle of training and emphasize it.

The remaining portions are active and not passive in their attempts to manipulate the opponent. Seal is simply blocking the opponent's movements so that the technique will work. This is another instance in which a simple visualization technique with emphasis on sealing will train in access to po. Unbalance must be used in conjunction with rooting. To unbalance someone requires that you be rooted and that you manipulate the opponent in some manner to take only his balance and not uproot him. If you uproot him then you relinquish other options. You uproot with intention, not by accident. The push is trained at the candle with visualizations and also in the form.

What is important is that you understand the nature of the training. It is not physical, but is instead a mental form of training in which it is the primitive portions of the mind with which you are dealing. You should have the overview of your training that it is multifaceted and all aspects impinge on your training. These different approaches are trained separately, but they actually overlap in the reality of the situation.

15-10 Hua Jing and Po

Hua jing operates exclusively within the domain of po. It is the most difficult internal aspect of the striking arts. Because there is no feedback within po, it is necessary to key on the absence of feedback to identify hua jing when it occurs. It is by default that you practice hua jing. It is by recognizing that something different has occurred and it was effortless, spontaneous and there was no feedback allowing you to discover how this occurred that you could discern hua jing.

By reducing the effort at an jing and with increased reliance on visualizations to move qi to the fingertips, you can determine whether it was a high level of an jing or hua jing that has occurred, and it will occur spontaneously. It is by recognizing it when it occurs and attempting to duplicate what occurred prior to it that we gain in hua jing. It is by the development from ming jing through an jing that we build pathways, the nine pearls and the visualizations that allow us move into this tenuous area.

If you are not song by the time you are attempting hua jing then you efforts will be fruitless.

Any effort other than maintaining stance and the almost imperceptible driving of the waist will place you in the domain of the yi mind. It is imperative that you do things with shen ming as your guiding principle. Shen ming is to do things naturally without thinking about it. The best example of shen ming is the play that occurs among children. It is spontaneous, fun, aggressive yet playful. We can take many of the elements within natural play and incorporate them within the training of hua jing. It is the enjoyment of play that makes it an effortless effort and natural in its occurrence. This can be included within the training of hua jing by virtue of the smile. It is difficult to be intensive, controlling and pre-eminent with a smile on your face. It is a long and arduous road to excel in hua jing. Every effort on your part, places you within the domain of the yi mind and not po. It is wei wu wei that must prevail. It is the "not doing" of the shaman. Not only must you act effortlessly and be song, but also it must be natural without thought and action must come out of inaction. This is a very high level of performance and cannot be taught in the same sense as fa jin. It is an individual effort in the same sense that you are alone in meditation, even as you are guided by a master, there is no one in there with you experiencing this inner life. This makes for a very lonely and courageous effort. It is by virtue of your mastery over your inner life that you can attain this level of performance.

The martial defensive aspects are covered by ming jing and an jing until hua jing is perfected. It is through this development path that hua jing is perfected. It is within the practice of the two lower forms of jing that hua jing will spontaneously occur. It is with the knowledge of the existence of hua jing and its characteristics that you create the possibility of its development. Without this knowledge your efforts would be stunted at the an jing level and there would be no pressure to reach a higher level.

An important and much misunderstood aspect of hua jing training is that of "not doing." If you are doing something with a purpose, or with the intent of gain, no matter how remote, then you are operating within the domain of the yi mind. Every aspect of training up to this point has been leading you to place the yi mind and po within close proximity so that there is visual communication between the two. The most difficult aspect of training is to utilize the yi mind to allow "not doing" to occur. You must train without the intention of personal gain. The training must include elements that are done without any possible personal gain or any redeeming feature. An example of this would be to leave one shoelace untied, or reverse the direction that you wear a belt. You must be imaginative in this. If you are deriving any satisfaction from doing this, then you must switch to something else. If you can preoccupy the yi mind with things that are not directed at its own personal gratification, the yi mind will then lose interest. We do not want a parallel existence between the yi mind and po, but rather for this instance in which hua jing occurs, we want our presence to be only within po. We do not want to remain within po therefore, we must key our attempts to occur only within the time period we are attempting hua jing. This can be done by tying hua jing and "not doing" together. It is by virtue of doing hua jing without doing hua jing that we gain in hidden force. It is wei wu wei that must be developed and this cannot be done with intent.

When you do hua jing at the lazhu, then it is necessary not to use muscular effort and to use visualizations of the technique. It is better to visualize the candle as getting brighter on the storage phase and going out on the emission stage. You would do this periodically during an jing training. The training overlaps until you have merged into training for hua jing. The simplest way to do this at the lazhu is practice being like a willow. This has most of the necessary ingredients if you do it without the intention of putting out the candle, and if you do it without the expectation of any gain.

15-11 Moving into Non-perceptive Space

The closer we get to po in our development of hua jing, the more we leave behind those landmarks that give us reassurance. We leave yiwan dongxi, the world of the ten thousand things, for something that for our word dominated sequential mind is utter chaos. A rigid demanding person that requires precision in definitions and logical statements would find this very disconcerting.

When you actually operate within the hua jing level of force there is a definite perceptual change in what you receive as sensory feedback. It is not entirely accurate to say that there is no feedback within po. You have the usual visual field, which is attended to in an abbreviated manner. The peripheral field is predominant, but when you operate in this arena and you are for instance in the middle of a throw, you will not see the individual but instead you will see a number of circular arcs of various colored light prescribing the path that the energy of movement is taking. Many advanced martial artist have reported this. It seems to be a device of po in transmitting whatever it is that it sees or it may very well be exactly what it sees. The point is that you should withhold your expectations and allow po to deliver to you its own perceptions.

Within the realm of the wisdom mind, you are attending to the ten thousand things and your attention is captivated. Perceptions are complex and conceptual. You have access to all kinds of associations and possibilities. Within the realm of po, everything is simplified down to the level of incoming and outgoing energy. Instead of conceptual thinking it is the manipulation of images that is paramount.

15-12 Inward and Outward Breathing Rhythms

If you use the breath as a means of coordinating the movements within techniques, this requires a stylization of the breathing sequence. In all cases, the inward inspiration of air must be assigned to the storage phase in ming jing and an jing levels of force and to the emission phase in hua jing. The outward or expiration phase assigned to the emission of energy or force in ming jing and an jing levels of force and to the storage phase in hua jing. The exhale must proceed and end before the release of qi in either technique or strike in both an jing and ming jing. Hua jing is the exception because of the need to compress the interval between the start and end of the inhaling and exhaling cycle. If you remember the difference between a fire and an explosion, then you know it is the time interval that makes the difference. This compression of the time interval in hua jing is derived from inserting an extended inhalation right before the release of fa jin. The exhale is merely a release from the inhale, but it is still an exhale. This then is the time compression required to yield the effortless explosive force of hua jing

It is within the water path that this reversal of energy flow and breathing occurs. Hua jing is a refinement of the earlier forms of expression of power. It is the final stage and maximum relaxation results from the inspiration right before release. It is virtually impossible to be tense on inhale. Tension is counterproductive to inhale, the bodies natural tendency is to be relaxed on inhale to keep from resricting the intake of air. To make this perfectly clear, when at the hua jing level of performance you must exhale on storage and inhale on emission of force. The release is a relaxed exhalation, which is unforced.

15-13 When is the Way Open

The yarrow sticks or bones were cast and read in primitive shamanistic Chinese society in order to determine if the way was open, or more properly, if one had access to the Tao. Access to the Tao required one to remove the yi mind and enter into the realm of po. If one was within this realm then access to the energies of qi and the ability to manipulate them and all it entailed was possible. The original purpose of the yarrow sticks was limited to this predictive capability and it worked well for that circumscribed objective. It was centuries later that it was altered into a complex discipline of prognostication and its effectiveness and force within the shamanistic culture changed.

In addition to the yarrow, there are many ways of predicting the opening of the way. It is essential to know whether the way is open, because in order to evaluate our progress in accessing po, we must have indicators other than tossing the yarrow for determining accessibility.

The sudden shock, which occurs when you are attacked, or you are in some kind of emergency results many times in a freezing of mental and physical activity, this is a direct result of the immediate departure of the yi mind. The yi or wisdom mind departs because it has access to past and future consequences. It can determine the outcome. It is fear that drives the yi mind to escape. This is one of the most important uses of the opening of the way. It is the initial fear of a confrontation that allows us to access po. This has already been discussed.

If there is a time dilation such that the movements of events around you have slowed remarkably, then the way is open. This is due to the accelerated effects of the po mind. It gives the appearance that everything else has slowed to a relatively high degree. This is a perceptual effect caused by the acceleration of action within the po mind because of its more direct method of action.

If you can affect tumo then the way is open. Tumo is the deliberate raising of the temperature of some part of the body through meditative practice, for instance the right hand while the left remains a normal temperature. If you can do this then the way is open.

If you sense a slow pulsing vibration within the body at about 2 to 5 cycles per second the delta cycle of brain wave research while you are awake, then access is there. This is simply conscious awareness when at the depths of the sleep cycle.

If in the midst of chaos you are calm and serene, then it is more than likely you have accessed po. It is axiomatic that the yi mind will not be calm and serene in the midst of chaos.

The aura or surround that is sometimes visible around living things is a good indicator that you are within po and not totally in the domain of the yi mind.

A non-verbal and nonlogical state of reverie is an indicator. Since po does not understand, anything beyond the eternal now and therefore cannot formulate any action, which derives information from the past and projects it into the future. Existence within the eternal now is evidence that the way is open.

Sensations of joint expansion or a sensation of popping within the joint are common meditative signposts and within the moving meditation of Taiji, they can also be an indicator.

Lowering of the pulse rate or blood pressure can be an indicator, since this is an autonomic function not under control of the yi mind.

The movement of the attention within the visual field from the fovea or clear vision portion of the visual field to the peripheral vision is a good indicator of the presence of po.

If animals and birds are not acting properly within your immediate vicinity, then it is conceivable that you are within po and the way is open.

One of the surest ways of being certain that the way is open is by the presence of the dragons's hum and the tiger's roar accompanied by the sense of vibrant activity within the body.

There are many more indicators, but this should suffice to gain a sense of the ways in which it is possible to determine if the way is open. It is of importance to know if the way is open since it is more effective to train po directly rather than affect it through the yi mind. These indicators work because the world we live in is interconnected in ways that are beyond our comprehension. Science is only beginning to realize how odd our existence is within this narrow slice of reality. To be enlightened is to be aware. It does not make you a better person or even a good one, only an aware one. It is true that the awareness can have survival value, but that is only over a large number of events. For the individual its survival potential is in its use in training the po mind.

Taiji places great emphasis on retraining the mind of the adept. It is not simply one of becoming yielding as many think, but it is by virtue of the access to po and the parallel existence between po and yi that the real gains are made. The sinusoidal wave of attention, moving from yi to po and back in a continuous cycle allows one to change the frequency of this wave cycle and keep the two within an interactive range. When it is stated that Taiji balances the mind-body relationship, it is this close proximity and interaction of the yi and po minds that is referenced. If you only understand this principle in Taiji, then your gains will be spectacular.

15-14 Zhen Zheng Ren

This is one of the avenues of advancement on the way to enlightenment by means of the study of the martial arts. It is not the fighting aspect of the martial arts that is of concern, but instead the generation of energy for martial purposes. The systematic development and storage of qi within the body is of paramount importance to those on the way to enlightenment. The immortal or real human being as the Chinese call an enlightened person is one who has no longer any need for yiwan dongxi or the ten thousand things. He has removed desire and the intent that interferes in the natural order of things (gui lu). He understands wei wu wei in its true Taoist sense and merely observes the world languishing in the three treasures (san bao) and san cai or three powers.

It is by removing himself from the turmoil of normal existence through stilling his mind and placing his attention on all existence that he rises above internal conflicts that plague most of us. By simply concerning himself with something other than his own personal existence, he has allowed himself to access a greater awareness and greater powers. It is also because of this greater awareness and separation from self interest that he has great power, yet this enormous power is of little use for someone who has little if any desire for the yiwan dongxi. He uses minimal energy in conflict with the outer world therefore has access to greater amounts, and in addition to moving from po to shen, he has chosen to be involved with humanity only to the extent that it will elevate humanity to the condition of zhen zheng ren and finally to the immortal (xian).

16

Lazhu Fangfa

16-1 Training Methodolgy

Lazhu fangfa is a means of assembling all the visualization techniques of Taiji under one umbrella. It is through visualizations of the yi mind and po that communication and cooperation can exist between the two. The sense of the opponent in doing the form, seeing the enemy at the candle, visualizing the opponent at interception practice with the soft ball fighting sequence and all other techniques are tied to the striking techniques in such a manner that it is not necessary to actually practice striking the attacking individual. The method that is utilized in training is unique. It is the mind that we are training and in many ways it is a retraining that occurs. The retraining must occur within the yi mind because it has to be trained to relinquish control and work in unison with po in an unusual nonlogical patterned and visual manner.

This is a complex reprogramming of responses to specific behavioral situations. It is not unlike the reprogramming of children in what is called patterning, in which the child is forced through a reprogramming from crawling stages using four people one on each arm and leg. The patterned movements are forced on the child over an hour's time for many weeks to impress on the brain the proper sequence of movements.

If you think in terms of the Taiji form as a patterned sequence and it in conjunction with the interception practice; candle practice; fighting sequence; walking the trigram and other practices as a means of retraining the yi mind and also training po: you will then have a good grasp of internal nature of Taiji. The fighting techniques of the internal arts are the same fighting techniques of the hard arts. It is the manner in which you handle incoming energy and execute the force employed in the techniques that is different. Taiji is not the same as a soft gong fu. Major differences occur and usually there is a merging with the opponent's forward motion not a soft block and the energy of the opponent is not stopped but allowed to continue and becomes a part of the offense. The actual difference lies in the mental visualizations and the movement of qi throughout the body in predetermined channels.

The slow movement of the form, although it does have many martial applications such as balance and strength enhancement, is essentially a mental training. It is because of its resemblance to the perceived time dilation that occurs within po during crisis situations that the slowness of the form has real benefit. It mimics this time dilation inducing shen to be within the state of po rather than the yi mind. Much of the inner nature of the internal arts is this duplication of events to approximate the actual natural occurrences so that wei-wu-wei may prevail and allow the events to occur. It takes considerable effort at not exerting an effort, if that makes any sense. This retraining of mental and physical reactions must be foremost in training. Even with extreme effort, it is difficult to reprogram behavior.

Most of the colorful language and eccentricities of training in the ancient martial arts occurred during a period of great illiteracy. The perpetuation of knowledge was in an oral tradition and a part of the indigenous culture. It is wrong to assume that we would share the same meaning from a translation of an ancient culture and language. We can understand much of the nuances of meaning that are involved in the training by determining what actually works and what does not.

The demands that can be placed on the student are much less in this culture and in this time. We do have an advantage in that we are dealing with a literate society and it is therefore possible to teach principles and accelerate the learning process. If we teach the underlying principles and their application, we can utilize visualizations in place of actual techniques. The movements within the mind train our muscle senses just as if we were actual doing the techniques without the exhausting training of the ancients.

16-2 Wei Wu Wei

The Taoist has an idiomatic expression, "The Tao does not act, yet there is nothing that it does not do." This expression is a central theme of Taoism. The concept of wei wu wei is the act of not doing. The expression is likely phrased in this way, because there is considerable thought about the paradox of wu wei. The expression itself is derived from the three characters in the I Ching as it was written by Lao Tzu. These three characters included in the I Ching are, wei, wu, and wei. The characters occur in this sequence in the I Ching. Direct transliteration of the Chinese characters into English yields the English concepts of action—non—-action and this appears to be a paradox since action and inaction comes from the attempts to discover how it is possible to arrive at action without any physical effort or action on one's part. The separation into wu-wei or non action is a contrived one. There is no non action separate from action. The paradox exists only in a philosophical sense if you separate the characters and only consider wu wei. Itwould be more accurate if it was stated as as action with non action. This paradox occurs because of the western civilizations cultural tendency to place the conclusion at the end of the discourse after a persuasive rationale in support of the stated premise and conclusion. It is in the cultural preference of the Chinese to place the premise and conclusion first and then establish the logical analysis at the end. Considering this structural sequence of thought, action is therefore a conclusion of the beginning premise of non action. It is then becomes necessary to interpret what the Taoist mean when they use the term non action.

The unnecessary outcome of this explanation is a restatement of the paradox that incorporates all the tenets of Taoism, but our interest is in the application of all these principles in a martial sense. The pertinence of non action exists within the interaction of the human nature (hun) and the animal nature (po).

The training in Taiji, as has been stated earlier, is mental more than it is physical. It is through the activity as it is conducted by the mind of po (the action portion) and perceived by the hun mind or the yi aspect of the hun mind, as having occurred without any activity on its part or (non action). This occurs because of the lack of feedback within the mind of po. It is possible that there is feedback within po, but that it is not transferred to the yi mind. In either case, the effect is that the perception within the yi mind is that action has occurred without effort or involvement of the yi mind. It is as if the action had occurred on its own. The paradox reflects this loss of feedback, which would render some causality to the activity. This is also reflected in the concept of jue xue, which means to stop the learning. It does not mean that you should cease educating yourself, but that the effort at training should be ceased and the action should be allowed to happen. As in most sports there comes a time in which the player no longer attempts to perform the activity, but instead does it automatically without thought. It is natural in that it flows with the activity and is non-contentious (bu zheng). To be non-contentious does not mean being non-combative. It means not forcing your intentions or desires on the situation. It means to allow it to unfold according the natural flow of things. These two things jue xue and bu zheng are conditions that invoke wei-wu-wei.

It is the intention within Taoism and Taiji to operate in life with wei-wu-wei predominant in thought and action. The Taoist do this through meditation and a sedentary, but active life, and the Taiji adept does this through the parallel training and the interacting of the yi mind and po.

16-3 Jue Xue

Jue xue means to give up learning, or more accurately, it means to go beyond learning. It is the endurance of intense long-term training that elicits jue xue. A time is reached within training schedules in which the mind is no longer required to participate directly in the regimen. The yi mind is no longer engaged in the training activity. This occurs in most intense activity in the martial arena, but to the Taoist this is a way of life. wei wu wei is a consequent philosophical strategy to the existential life of the Taoist and the Taiji adept as a Taoist in creating this inner and outer harmony that is a mental aspect of their way of life. A Taoists stops the process of learning by going beyond the process and all forms or distinctions between yin and yang are reduced to nothingness (kong kong ji hua gui wu you). It is not that they stop educating themselves, as education is considered essential and an important part of their lives. They remove themselves from learning as a process by acting without concern for themselves. They do things without concern for gain. Taoist do not educate themselves to acquire the benefits of society and all it will bring them, but so that they may advance the condition of man. It is this quiet perception of the realm of the eternal now and this merging of yin and yang into one that they seek.

16-4 Pu

Utter simplicity is all that characterizes the Taost philosophy. This concept exemplifies Taoist thought. In the martial arena, they routinely control the opponent with a serene, calm demeanor that does not do justice to the strength of their resolve. It is not with some elaborate manipulative technique that they opt to defeat an aggressive individual, but instead they merely let them move effortlessly into emptiness only to be confused when they become aware of their failed strategy. This typically leaves the aggressor confused and destroys their offensive strategy, and this is typically more in harmony with their concepts of bu zheng or to be non-contentious. They constantly seek to to avoid the impulsive, chaotic and aggressive behaviors of others, and interact with them only in the sense of elevating their existence.

The ying er or infant contains the youthful innocence of the young child. It is the absence of experience and lack of social nuance that epitomizes it. It lacks knowledge of fame or fortune, shame or guilt or embarrassment. It does not comprehend the concept of sin. The ying er may unintentionally injure or offend another, but there is never a malicious intent. The infant is the embodiment of pure innocence and emptiness. It is the esoteric mirror polished and reflecting perfectly and it is that which we search for in Taiji practices.

Pu can be thought of as the uncarved block of wood in the raw state, unaltered, and not marked by the vagaries of life. By way of entering into into this unfinished and raw state that wei wu wei and all else becomes possible. Ziran is then possible, and we arrive at a state of self-so, a spontaneous state of existence that is natural in performance and is the fundamental priciple that the tao follows on its evolutionary path. The Taiji adept must then strive to follow this precept and return to this simplest of existence. It is important for lazhu fangfa that you do not strive to put out the candle. It is intention on your part that will cause you difficulty. Desire and intent will lead you away from the tao toward the controlling aspects of hun and the yi mind. There is much Taoism in the current expression "just do it."

16-5 Qi Qi Guai Guai

This translates as making strange things happen. Much has been said about avoiding powers of the mind, not that there is anything inherently bad or dangerous about them. This caution exists in the same sense that there is a danger in the the ten thousand things. If you are captivated by them, then your training is stilted and you never reach the ultimate in your art. The danger does not lie in the area of qi qi guai guai, but instead within the area of desire and intent. If you are captivated by some object and some emotion, then you have not and cannot relinquish desire and intent and therefore you cannot still the mind and acquire the water path method, which is the Taoist method of obtaining enlightenment. It is all right to acquire and to use qi qi guai guai, but not for personal gain. In the aid of your fellow man or in the interest of the sage person to promote the well fare and level of attainment of the average person, then it is perfectly acceptable. It is also unacceptable to use your martial knowledge for personal gain. Again, it is perfectly acceptable in the service of humankind. It is unacceptable in the sense that it will prevent you from obtaining your goal of hua jing.

16-6 Hua Jing and the Water Path

The main objective of lazhu fangfa is to train the Taiji adept in both the soft jings of fa jin and the water method of developing maximum force as in hua jing. The water method is the approach utilized by the Taoist. Buddhism and Confucianism are mostly concerned with the fire path. Others use a combination of fire path and water path to accomplish this, and this offers a means of distinguishing them from the Taoist. Taoism supports the water path as a device in acquiring enlightenment.

The water path is not an easy path especially in regard to wei-wu-wei. It is difficult to breach this gap between the abstract mental concepts of the idea so that you can arrive at action from inaction without the actual act itself. Mental concepts are easy to accept, but to put it into practice is much more difficult.

Practicing hua jing or perfect force (wei-wu-wei) at the candle requires that you begin with ming jing (hidden force) in which by now you have become relatively proficient, and move from the fire path to the water path. This is the reverse flow of qi in meditation and fa jin. Instead of flowing from the Tantien down to the hui yin then up to the ming men through the yu zhen, across the bai hui, down the shang tantien to return to the qi hai or Tantien, the flow is reversed and movement is upward from the tantien to the Shang tantien down the yu zhen to the ming men, through the hui yin and upward to the tantien. Once you start on the water path, you must remain there to avoid losing progress. It has to be a constant and concerted effort to remain on the path or you will revert to the fire path when attacked and your hua jing will not be evident. You must lose intent and desire and by centering your thoughts on the tantien and merely allow the candle to go out. If you engage in any form of yi mind function then it will not be effective. This begins with a refinement of an jing when you have reached that level in which there is very little movement in emitting an jing and it is seemingly effortlessly executed. There is, however, a muscular component, and this must be gradually removed and the flow of qi eventually becomes the movement of the yi mind through the reverse path. For hua jing the reverse flow path is short circuited at the Tantien and allowed to flow to the emitting extremity. This then will become with long and arduous practice xue jue and the flow of hua jing will occur when necessary without effort on your part. You will then be ziran.

16-7 You Xing Zhie Shi Jia, Wu Xing Fang Wei Zhen

This transliterates as "have form is false, no form is correct direction." The ultimate in the internal martial art is to move from the formal and stylized to the transitory, not merely for the enlightening aspects of it, but for considerable martial reasons. This is the highest level of performance in any martial arena. It embodies all the principles of Taiji and all the principles of Taoism. You do not need to be a Taoist to do Taiji, but you do need to adhere to the principles of Taoism to master Taiji.

It is not necessary to compromise your opponent totally to be successful. The level of your performance is determined by your ability to handle the opponent without harming or destroying him. It is one in which you teach him by example to be a better person a sage person.

Taiji becomes something else other than a martial art. It is a way of life that takes on an existence of its own. All of your life experiences become a part of this ancient mind you have created. Even at this stage of the game, you will not know the full range of your capabilities unless you have had an actual encounter that verifies you training. It is your faith in the training you have undertaken that sustains you. All of those forces of nature that are possible through po will serve to protect you without you actively seeking them. They will coalesce around the ancient mind and only emerge when you are threatened. If you are unsure of your ability to contend, it is a good thing. The alternative is a contentious person, who is out to prove himself through his martial capabilities. If you never have to use them, then you are very fortunate. The surprising thing about Taiji on this level is that nothing surprises you. If you have attained a high level with your feeble efforts, just think of the capabilities of a sage person who has devoted his life to this under an extremely capable teacher. Think for a moment and try to determine how you would fight someone who has no form, no techniques and is not attempting to destroy you. How devastating is it to fight someone who has no concern for the fight and views it as merely an inconvenience? This is the true Taiji, the Taiji of the sage person. It exists on a level that few of us will ever attain. Make no mistake, even those that appear to be well accomplished may not even be aware of this level and merely give lip service to it.

Remember to be bu zheng or non-contentious and you will have no form. You xing zhie shi jia, wu xing fang wei zhen.

Glossary

Ancient Mind	This is the warrior mind of po. It exists in the eternal now and it does not know fear. It is the primitive mind, the mind of trance-like states. The trance occurs because the ancient mind is typically untrained and therefore unresponsive.
An Jing	Hidden force, the second level of internal energy development. This level is characterized by the diminishment of external visible movement. This is an energy pulse delivered to the opponent when the point of application is already in contact with the opponent. It is the same force as fa jin and generated in the same manner.
Bai Hui	The crown point at the top of the head known as the hundred meetings. It belongs to the governing vessel. It is called tailing in the martial arts of the Taoist school.
Beautiful Lady's Hand	The graceful curvature of the arm, forearm and hand that stores energy within this curvature. The energy is released through the straightening of the curvature. It is also called jade lady's hand.
Blade Hand	Jim Ji, which is striking with the bottom edge of the hand.
Bu Zheng	To be non-contentious.
Chakra	Hindu for centers of an external energy source that terminates in the body. There is a transfer of energy from the world of shen into the body through the chakras. This is a visual representation of the energy system that po presents to the yi mind.
Cha'n	This is the original term for Zen of Japan that was borrowed from the Chinese.
Chan Sichou	Silk reeling or the storage of energy within the body from the twisting of muscle and tendons. It also refers to the threading of qi through the body. It is also a term for the coiling techniques of Taiji.
Chen Jen	Immortal, not ruled by what he sees.

Ch'ien (Qian)	The creative masculine principle. One f the two forces that characterize the change of the dichotomy formed from the tao. It is active in character.
Chin Hua (Jin Hua)	The Golden Flower or the experiencing of the Golden Light of Illumination.
Closing	This is a movement of the torso such that raising the shoulders and hollowing the chest in conjunction with moving the rounded arms closer together creates storage of energy. Closing can also be used as a release of energy created by the opening movement.
Conception Vessel	Ren Mei or the front vessel for movement of qi through the body.
Cranial Pump	A line forward of the top of the ears which can be felt when the teeth are clenched. The compression of the muscles in this area strengthens the upward pulse.
Double weighting	The even distribution of weight on both legs. It is considered a fault in Taiji.
Dragon's Hum and Tiger's Roar	Ear sounds similar to tinnitus as a result of the way being open. Dragon's hum is the sound in the right ear and tiger's roar is in the left ear. It is an indication the way is open.
Du Mei	The governing vessel at the back of the torso running from the hui yin point to the point on the top of the head where it merges with the ren mei point.
Eternal Now	Existence within the moment such that there is no past or future.
Fa Jin	The striking force of Taiji using internal energy.
Fang Song Gong	The method of relaxed effort.
Gate of Life	The ming men or point on the body posterior to the sternum which is essentially the hollow of the back.
Governing Vessel	The ren mei vessel or the energy path at the front of the torso.
Golden Bell Cover	Surrounding the body with a cover of protective qi that serves as a defense against external force.
Gui Lu	The natural order of the things.
Hu Kou	Tiger's mouth, the area between the thumb and index finger.
Hua Jing	Perfect force, the third level of internal energy development.
Hui Huo	Hidden method.

Hsing	Human nature.
Hui Yin	The point on the base of the spine in the perineum that is a difficult passage for qi.
Hun	It encompasses the world of the ten thousand things and is a product of xing. The wisdom mind yi and the emotional mind xin are a part of it.
Huo Banye	Living midnight, the void that is not empty, also the hours between eleven and one at night. This also can refer to the precursor to the Golden Flower (the black void).
Jade Pillow	Yuzhen, a point on the occipital area of the skull. This is one of the difficult passages of qi in its movement throughout the body. It is where your head makes contact with the pillow.
Jing	The energy of force generated by internal means as opposed to the use of muscles(li) of the external styles.
Jiu Zenzhu	Nine Pearls or the firm connection of the joints to create a pathway for the storage and emission of jing.
Jue Xue	First relinquish ignorance then relinquish learning. Stop learning and just do it.
Kun	The receptive feminine principle. One of the forces that characterize change or the dichotomy formed from the tao. It is yielding or passive in character.
Lazhu Fangfa	The candle method of Taiji or the utilization of a candle (lazhu) for training purposes.
Living Midnight	A Taoist term for the mind in a state of complete stillness in which the blackness of the void is visible. It is entering the dark door or the empty chamber.
Local Qi	Qi that is derived from the local energy stored within the muscle groups being used. It is only a temporary storage and not an accumulation of qi.
Ma Pu	Also ma bu stance or the horse stance. Used by martial artist for leg strengthening and endurance. It assists in developing internal storage of energy.
Ming	this is the life process identified with the animal side of existence. It is fate and the primitive elements of existence. Po is formed from its essence.
Ming Jing	Visible force, the first level of internal development.

Ming Men	A point on the back just behind the sternum where the internal energy can be moved either upward or outward to be expressed in the hands as fa jing or an jing.
Nei Shi Gongfu	Internal perception gongfu. When you can feel the internal movement of qi and can distribute it to the organs, then you have nei shi gongfu. It is the gongfu of internal vision.
Nine Bends in the Pearl	A Chinese term used to indicate the difficulty in threading the qi through various difficult passages in the body.
Nine Pearls	Jiu zhenzhu, this is the joints of the body which are made firm in order to assist in the passage of qi for martial purposes.
Old Ox power	Jiu gongniu jing, the rotation of the waist such that the lead right arm is rotating counter clockwise, and the left lead arm is rotating clockwise.
Opening	This is a movement of the torso such that the energy stored on closing is released by the outward movement of the rounded arms. It also can serve as a means of storage of energy.
Pedagogic Imagery	Vivid imagery from the realm of po which has some value in the learning process.
Po	This is the product of ming. It is the primitive mind, the mind of the reptilian brain stem. It is involved in bodily processes and it can be trained to perform functions specific to the martial arts. It is the ancient mind.
Qi Belt	The area of the waist at the belt line where it is difficult t move the qi for fa jin or the universal circulation.
QiGong	An internal and external form of exercise derived from the ancient da wu or great dance of ancient China.
Reh Qi	This is the warmth or heat generated in the body, it is the same as the tumo of the Tibetans. It also can mean that a person is alive, in that he has body heat.
Ren Mei	This is the red line or conception vessel at the front of the body. It goes from the hui yin to the top of the head traveling up the front side of the body.
Reverse Taoist Breathing	This is a form of breathing in which the abdomen is contracted inward and downward on nhale and released on exhale. It is expressly used for generating qi and in the use of fa jin and an jing.
Sacral Pump	The sacral pump is the sacrum which when contracted in the energy cycle assists the movement of qi across the pelvic girdle.

San Bao	The three treasures, jing or essence, qi or energy, shen of spirit.
San Cai	The three powers, Heaven, Earth, and Man
Secret Sword Hand	Gim Ji, the extension of the index and middle fingers with the others folded under the thumb. This serves energy distribution and also serves as a weapon in sword fighting when the second weapon is lost.
Shen	The spirit body of the human condition.
Shen Ming	Mind understanding, it is to do something naturally without thinking.
Sheng Jen	Saintly man, divinely inspired and intuitively wise.
Substantial Leg	The leg that contains most of the weight distribution in a stance or posture.
Shang Tantien Celestial Eye	the space between the eyebrows, also the upper elixer field or upper tantien.
Song	A relaxed sentience that involves also relaxing the vaso-constrictors.
Taiji Tu	Taiji yin, yang symbol.
Ta Chuan	The Great Treatise or a precursor to the I Ching.
Tai Yi Jin Hua Congshi	the secret of the golden flower.
Taiji Sphere	This is a visualization exercise. It requires imagining the body performing as a sphere in which it contacts the earth at one point only and moves as a ball does when touched.
Tantien	Lower tantien, sea of qi, or qi hai, the energy center just below the umbilical cord, and three inches inward.
Ten Thousand Things	Yiwan dongxi, or the myriad of things making up the phenomena world.
Threading the Qi	Moving the qi through the difficult passages.
Tiao Xin	Regulating the mind, when large tao is taught, first stop thought, then thought of no thought.
Tien Hsia	The world of humanity or "all under heaven." This includes earth and humanity.
Ting Jing	Listening energy or sensing the movement of the opponent.
Tumo	Generating heat within the body through visualization techniques.
Warrior Mind	The ancient mind or po. The primitive reptilian mind, the brain stem.

Wisdom Mind	That aspect of hun that has logical properties.
Whole Body Power	The exertion of force with the accumulative force of unified movement of the body.
Wu Wei	Action without movement or the internalization of the source of fa jin. If you can create an emptiness or a void within you, the the tao may be able to fill this void.
Xia Qi	Killing air, or the use of posture or facial expression with loud vocalization to intimidate the opponent.
Xiao Cho Tien	Small universe circulation, from the tantien to hui yin, the mingmen, yuzhen, bai hui and the back to the tantien.
Xiao Tantien	Sea of qi, the lower tantien.
Xiao Xing Xing	Small star, or the point on the palm of the hand that is the end point of the long bones in the forearm. It is the point of contact in a palm strike. This is also the end point of the pericardial meridian.
Xin	The heart, the Chinese often use the heart in reference to the mind. The heart is considered the seat of the mind, especially the emotional mind.
Xu jin	Storing jin within the body.
Yang	Literally means the sunny side of the hill.
Yi Shou Tan Tien	Keeping the attention on the tantien. Literally, minds hand tantien.
Yin	Literally means the shady side of the hill. It is the inactive principle, the dark passive nature of things.
Yi Ting Shi	Stilling the Mind.
Yiwan Dongxi	The ten thousand things. This is the known world or the material world.
Yi Yi Yin Qi	Use your mind (wisdom mind) to lead your qi.
Yongchuan Point	A point in the center of the ball of the foot.
Yun Jin	To move jin through the body.
Yuzhen	Jade pillow, a point at the base of the skull or the occipital area.
Zhan Zhuang	Qi gong exercise standing like a tree or embracing the tree.
Zhen Jing	Whole body power.
Zhenzheng Ren	True or genuine person, an immortal.

| Zhong Din | Central balance or strength, maintaining root and balance through out the form and all movement. |
| Zhong Tantien | Upper tantien, the area between the brow. |

978-0-595-45157-9
0-595-45157-8

LaVergne, TN USA
14 February 2010
173039LV00001B/142/A